CW01180384

The Newtonian System of Philosophy Adapted to the Capacities of Young Gentlemen and Ladies. ... Being the Substance of six Lectures Read to the Lilliputian Society, by Tom Telescope, A.M. and Collected and Methodized ed 7

Frontispiece.

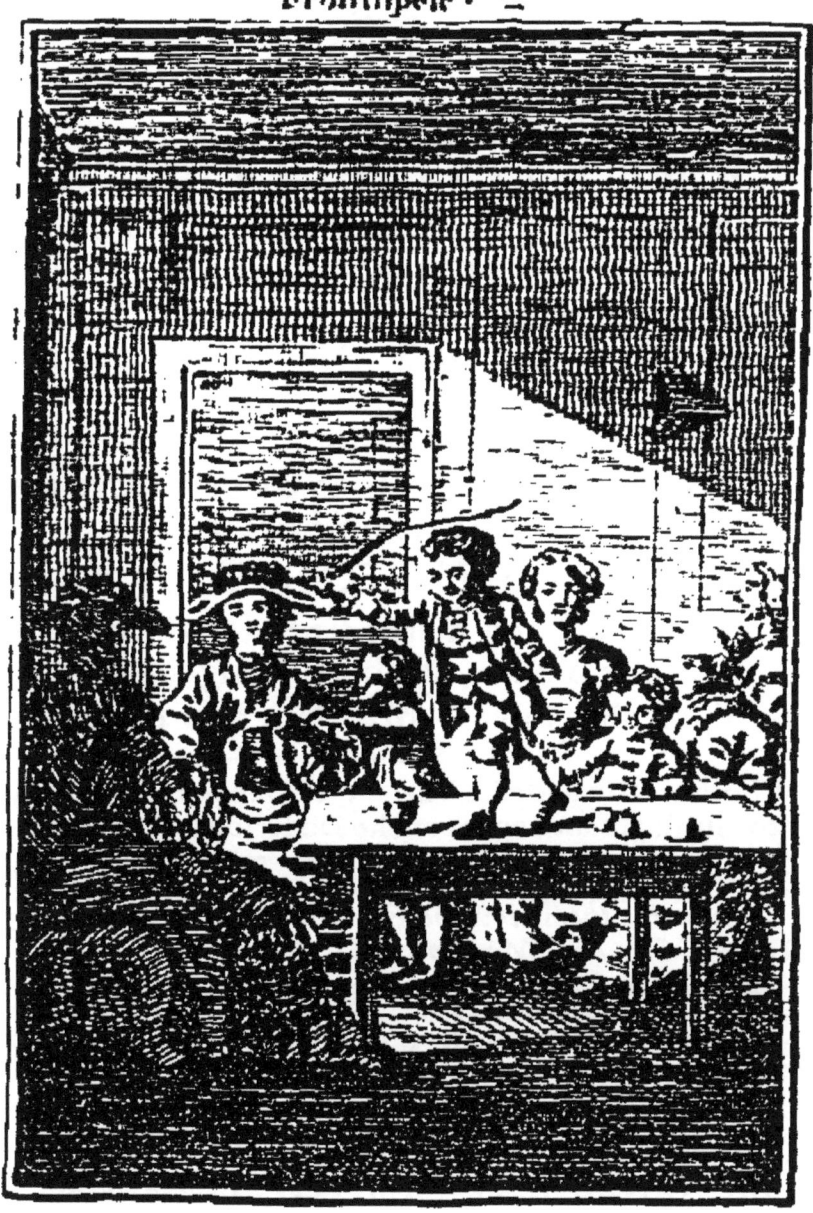

Lecture on Matter & Motion.

THE NEWTONIAN SYSTEM OF PHILOSOPHY

Adapted to the Capacities of Young GENTLEMEN and LADIES.

And familiarized and made entertaining by Objects with which they are intimately acquainted:

BEING

The Substance of SIX LECTURES read to the LILLIPUTIAN SOCIETY,

By TOM TELESCOPE, A.M.

And collected and methodized for the Benefit of the Youth of these Kingdoms,

By their old Friend MR. NEWBERY, in *St Paul's Church Yard.*

Who has also added a Variety of Copper Plate Cuts to illustrate and confirm the Doctrines advanced.

O Lord, how manifold are thy Works! In Wisdom hast thou made them all: the Earth is full of thy Riches. Young Men and Maidens, old Men and Children, praise the Lord   PSALMS.

THE SEVENTH EDITION.

LONDON.

Printed for T. CARNAN, (Successor to Mr J. NEWBERY) in *St Paul's Church Yard.*

MDCCLXXXVII

[Price One Shilling and Six-pence.]

TO THE
YOUNG GENTLEMEN and LADIES
OF
Great-Britain and *Ireland*,
THIS
PHILOSOPHY of TOPS and BALLS
Is humbly inscribed,
By their most obedient Servant,
J. NEWBERY.

✣✣✣✣✣✣✣✣✣✣✣✣✣✣

CONTENTS.

INTRODUCTION, page 1.

LECTURE I. *Of* MATTER *and* MOTION.
The Laws of Motion, page 5. Attraction *and* Gravitation, 9. *Figure of the* Earth, ib. Magnet *or* Loadstone, 12. *The Sphere of* Attraction, *and of* Repulsion, ib. Cohesion, ib. Electricity, 14.

LECTURE II. *Of the* UNIVERSE, *and particularly of the* SOLAR SYSTEM.
The Horizon, 18. Fixed Stars, 20. *The* Sun, *the* Planets, *and* Comets, 23. Eclipses *of the* Sun *and* Moon, 26. Motion *of the* Earth, 28. *Velocity* of Light, 31.

CONTENTS.

LECTURE III. *Of the* AIR, ATMOSPHERE, *and* METEORS.

The Four Elements, 34. Air, *and* Atmosphere, 37. *Elasticity of the* Air, 38. Wind-Gun, 40. Earthquakes, 41 Water, 42. Light *and* Sound, ib. Echo, 43. Air-Pump, 44. Ventilators, 48 Winds, 49. Mists, Fogs, *and* Clouds, 52. Rain, 53. Thunder, *and* Lightning, 55, 60. Snow, *and* Hail, 56. Northern Lights, 57. Jack-with-a-Lantern, *or* Will-with-the-Wisp, 58. Rainbow, 59. Halos, 60

LECTURE IV. *Of* MOUNTAINS, SPRINGS, RIVERS, *and the* SEA.

Mountains, 63 *Burning* Mountains, 68. Springs, 72. Rivers, 74. Lakes, ib. *The* Sea, 75. Tides, 76.

LECTURE V. *Of* MINERALS, VEGETABLES, *and* ANIMALS.

Earths, 79. Sand, Gravel, Chalk, *and* Rocks, ib. Fossils, 80. *Vulgar and precious* Stone, ib. Salts, 81. Mineral Substances, ib. Plants, 83. Animals, 90. Men, ib. Brutes, 91.

LECTURE VI. *Of the five Senses of* MAN, *and of his* UNDERSTANDING.

Origin of our Ideas, 100. Seeing, 103. Telescopes, 19, 106. *Separating Colours by the* Prism, 107. Hearing, 108. Smelling, 110. Tasting, 111. Touching, 114. Heat, *and* Cold 115. Pleasure, *and* Pain, 117. *Of the* Understanding, 119.

INTRODUCTION:

Being the Substance of

A LETTER to the Hon. ****.

DEAR SIP,

I AM desired by the Marchioness of *Setstar* to give you some account of those young Gentlemen and Ladies whom you saw enter the saloon the morning you left us, and who came to his Lordship's seat on an adventure the most extraordinary and the most to be admired of any I ever knew. You may remember it was holiday time, and these little gentry being come from school met first at the Countess of *Twilight's* to divert themselves; where they were so divided in their taste for amusements, that warm debates ensued. One proposed *Threading the Needle*, another *Hot-Cockles*, a third *Shuttle-cock*, a fourth *Blind-Man's-Buff*, and

INTRODUCTION.

at last *Cards* were mentioned. Master *Telescope*, a young gentleman of distinguished abilities, sat silent, and heard all with complacency and good temper till this diversion was proposed; but then he started from his seat, and begged they would think of some more innocent amusement. Playing at cards for money, says he, is so nearly allied to covetousness and cheating, that I abhor it; and have often wondered, when I was at *Bath* with my papa, how people, seemingly of years of discretion, could so far mistake themselves, and abandon common sense, as to lead a young *urchin* just breeched, or a little *doddle my-lady* in hanging sleeves, up to a gaming table, to play and bet for shillings, crowns, and perhaps guineas, among a circle of sharpers. Parents, continued he, might almost as well teach their children to thieve as to game; for they are kindred employments, and generally terminate in the ruin of both fortune and character. Lady *Twilight*, who is no friend to the modern modes of education, smiled at this young gentleman's remark, and desired him to point out some diversion himself. 'Tis impossible for me, Madam, says he, to find out an amusement suitable to the taste of the company, unless I was perfectly acquainted

with

with their dispositions; but were I to chuse, I should prefer those which not only divert the mind, but improve the understanding: and such are many of the diversions at the school where I am placed. We often play at *sham Orations, comical Disputes, measuring of Land and Houses, taking the Heights and Distances of Mountains and Steeples, solving Problems and Paradoxes, on Globes and Maps*, and sometimes at *Natural Philosophy*, which I think is very entertaining, and at the same time extremely useful; for whether our knowledge is acquired by these amusemens, and reading little books, or by serious and elaborate study, what is obtained will be equally serviceable. nay, perhaps that which is acquired in the entertaining manner may have the advantage; for, as it is conveyed to the mind with a train of pleasing ideas, it will be the more permanent and lasting, and the easier called up by the memory to our assistance.

The Countess was very desirous of knowing what sort of diversion could be made of Natural Philosophy: and finding her young visitors in the same disposition, she conducted them to the Marquis of *Setstar's*, that they might have the use of proper instruments. As my Lord Marquis was engaged in

company,

company, Lady *Twilight*, though nearly related to his Lordſhip, would not diſturb him, but led them through the ſaloon into a private parlour, where our little Philoſopher, at the requeſt of her Ladyſhip, immediately opened the Lecture, without making idle excuſes, or waiting for further ſolicitations, which he knew would be ill manners.

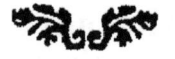

LECTURE I.

Of MATTER *and* MOTION.

BY *Matter*, my dear friends, *we mean the substance of all things*, or that of which all bodies are composed, in whatever form or manner they may present themselves to our senses: for this top, *Tom Wilson*'s ivory ball, the hill before us, that orange on the table, and all things you see, are made of matter differently formed.

As to *Motion*, I may save myself and you the trouble of explaining that, for every boy who can whip his top knows what motion is as well as his master.

Matter, or *Body, is indifferent to motion or rest.* As for example, now I whip my top, and it runs round, or is in motion; but when I no longer whip it, the top falls down, as you see, and is at rest.

When a body is in motion, as much force is required to make it rest, as was required while it was at rest, to put it in motion. Thus suppose a boy strikes a trap-ball with one hand, and another stands close by to catch it with one of his hands, it will require as much strength or force to stop that ball,

or

or put it in a state of rest, as the other gave to put it in motion, allowing for the distance the two boys stand apart.

No body or part of matter can give itself either motion or rest. and therefore a body at rest will remain so for ever, unless it be put in motion by some external cause; and a body in motion will move for ever, unless some external cause stops it.

This seemed so absurd to Master *Wilson*, that he burst into a loud laugh. What, says he, shall any body tell me that my hoop or my top will run for ever, when I know by daily experience that they drop, of themselves, without being touched by any body? At which our little Philosopher was angry, and having commanded silence: Don't expose your ignorance, *Tom Wilson*, for the sake of a laugh, says he; if you intend to go through my Course of Philosophy, and to make yourself acquainted with the nature of things, you must prepare to hear what is more extraordinary than this. When you say that nothing touched the top or the hoop, you forget their friction or rubbing against the ground they run upon, and the resistance they meet with from the air in their course, which is very considerable though it has escaped your notice. Somewhat

what too might be said on the gravity and attraction between the top or the hoop, and the earth; but that you are not yet able to comprehend, and therefore we shall proceed in our Lecture.

A body in motion will always move on in a straight line, unless it be turned out of it by some external cause. Thus we see that a marble shot upon the ice, if the surface be very smooth, will continue its motion in a straight line, till it is put to rest by the friction of the ice and air, and the force of attraction and gravitation.

The swiftness of motion is measured by distance of place, and the length of time in which it is performed. Thus if a cricket-ball and a fives-ball move each of them twenty yards in the same time, their motions are equally swift; but if the fives-ball move two yards while the cricket-ball is moving one, then is the motion of the fives-ball twice as swift as the other.

But the quantity of motion is measured by the swiftness of motion as above described, and the quantity of matter moved, considered together. For instance, if the cricket-ball be equal in bulk and weight to the fives-ball, and move as swift, then it hath an equal quantity of motion. But if the cricket ball

be

be twice as big and heavy as the fives-ball, and yet move equally swift, it hath double the quantity of motion, and so in proportion.

All bodies have a natural tendency, attraction, or gravitation towards each other. Here *Tom Wilson*, again laughing, told the company that Philosophy was made up of nothing but hard words. That is because you have not sense enough to enquire into, and retain the signification of words, says our Philosopher. All words, continued he, are difficult till they are explained; and when that is done, we shall find that gravity or gravitation will be as easily understood as praise or commendation, and attraction as easily as correction, which you deserve, *Tom Wilson*, for your impertinence.

Gravity, my dear friends, *is that universal disposition of matter which inclines or carries the lesser part towards the centre of the greater part; which is called* weight *or gravitation in the lesser body, but* attraction *in the greater, because it draws, as it were, the lesser body to it.* Thus all bodies on or near the earth's surface have a tendency, or seeming inclination, to descend towards its middle part or centre; and but for this principle in nature, the earth (considering its form and situation in the universe) could not subsist as it is, for we all suppose the earth

Of MATTER and MOTION.

earth to be nearly round, (nay, we are sure it is so, for my Lord *Anson*, and many other gentlemen, you know, have sailed round it) and as it is suspended in such a mighty void or space, and always in motion, what should hinder the stones, water, and other parts of matter falling from the surface, but the almighty arm of God, or this principle or universal law in nature, of attraction and gravitation, which he has established to keep the universe in order. To illustrate and explain what I have said, let us suppose the following figure to be the earth and seas. Let *Tom Wilson* stand at this point of the globe or earth where we are,

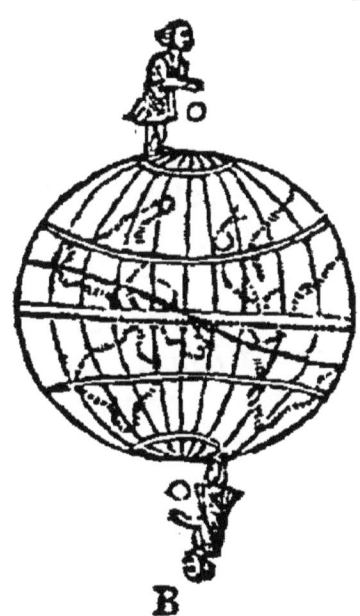

B

and

and *Hal Thompson* at the opposite part of the the earth, with his feet (as they must be) towards us: if *Tom* drop an orange out of his hand, it will fall down towards *Hal*: and if *Hal* drop an orange, it will fall seemingly upwards (if I may so express myself) towards *Tom*. and if these oranges had weight and power sufficient to displace the other particles of matter of which the earth is composed. so as to make way to the centre, they would there unite together and remain fixed and they would then lose their power of gravitation, as being at the centre of gravity, and unable to fall, and only retain in themselves the power of attraction.

This occasioned a general laugh; and *Tom Wilson* starting up, asked how Master *Thompson* was to stand with his feet upwards, as here represented, without having any thing to support his head? Have patience, says the little Philosopher, and I will tell you: but pray behave with good manners, Master *Wilson*, and don't laugh at every thing you cannot comprehend. This difficulty is solved, and all the seeming confusion which you apprehend of bodies flying off from each other is removed, by means of this attraction and gravitation

tion. Ask any of the sailors who have been round the world, and they will tell you that the people on the part of the globe over-against us do not walk upon their heads, though the earth is round; and though their heels are opposite ours, they are in no more danger of falling into the mighty space beneath them, than we are of falling (or rather rising I must call it here) up to the moon or the stars.

But besides this general law of attraction and gravitation, which effects all bodies equally and universally, there are particular bodies that attract and repel each other, as may be seen by the *Magnet* or *Loadstone*, which has not only the property of directing the needle of the mariner's compass, when touched with it, to the north; but also of attracting or bringing iron to it with one end, and repelling or forcing it away with the other end and *Sam Jones*'s knife, which was whet on a loadstone some years ago, still retains the power you see of picking up needles and small pieces of iron.

Glass, *Sealing Wax*, *Amber*, and *Precious Stones*, when chafed or rubbed till they are warm, will likewise both attract and repel feathers, hairs, straw, &c. which is sufficient

cient to prove that each of these bodies has a sphere of attraction assigned it, beyond which it will repel the same body it would otherwise attract.

When bodies are so attracted by each other as to be united or brought into close contact, they then adhere or cohere together, so as not to be easily separated, and this is called in Philosophy the *Power* of *Cohesion*, and is undoubtedly that principle which binds large bodies together; for all large bodies are made up of atoms or particles inconceivably small. And this cohesion will be always proportioned to the number of particles or quantity of the surface of bodies that come into contact or touch each other, for those bodies that are of a spherical form will not adhere so strongly as those that are flat or square, because they can only touch each other at a certain point; and this is the reason why the particles of water and quicksilver, which are globular or round, are so easily separated with a touch, while those of metals and some other bodies are not to be parted but with great force. To give us a familiar instance of this cohesion of matter, our Philosopher took two leaden balls, and filing a part off each, so that the two flat parts might come

into

into close contact, he gently pressed them together, and they united so firmly, that it required considerable force to get them asunder.

One thing I must tell you of magnetism, which seems pretty extraordinary. Master *Brown* took his uncle's sword, and supported it with the point downwards, by resting the shell of the hilt on the top of his two forefingers; and Master *Smith* was placed with his father's amber headed cane at about three or four feet distance, where he kept rubbing the amber head round on his waistcoat. After some little time the sword began to move, though at that distance; and some time after that it turned quite round; but was soon turned back again by Master *Smith*'s rubbing the amber head backwards, or in a contrary direction.

But what seems most worthy of our admiration is the Electrical Fire, which so plentifully abounds in the universe, and which is excited or made visible, by the friction or rubbing of a glass globe. This fire, by a very simple machine, may be conveyed into the human body, every part of which it pervades in an instant, and is said to be very serviceable in the cure of some disorders. It may be drawn from the ladies

ladies eyes, yet leaves them no less briliant than they were before. It may be drawn from thunder clouds, and is probably the same species of fire with the lightning, for Professor *Richmann* of *Hamburgh*, who fixed a machine to bring it down from the clouds in large quantities, was killed by the stroke it gave him.

The same force applied to two different bodies will always produce the same quantity of motion in each of them. To prove this, we put Master *Jones* into a boat, which (including his own weight) weighed ten hundred, on the *Thames* by the *Mill-Bank*; and on the *Lambeth* side, just opposite, we placed another boat (of one hundred weight) with a string tied to it. This string Master *Jones* pulled in the other boat; and we observed that as the boats approached each other, the small boat moved ten feet for every foot the other moved: which proves what we have before observed as to the quantity of motion.

Attraction is the stronger, the nearer the attracting bodies are to each other; and in different distances of the same bodies it decreases as the squares of the distance between the centres of those bodies increase. For if two bodies at a given distance attract each other

Of Matter and Motion.

other with a certain force, at half the distance they will attract each other with four times that force. But this I shall further explain in my next course of Lectures.

Two bodies at a distance will put each other in motion by the force of Attraction or Gravitation. This we know to be true by experience, though we cannot account for it; and therefore it is to be received as a principle in Natural Philosophy.

Here Master *Wilson*, again interrupting him, said that could not be true: for if two bodies at any distance could put one another in motion by their power of attraction, the earth and the moon would move towards each other in a straigth line, and unite; and then, says he, laughing, all Dr *Wilkins*'s machines for flying thither would be useless

But you should consider, says the Philosopher, if a body, that by the attraction of another would move in a straight line towards it, receives a new motion any ways oblique to the first, it will no longer move in a straight line, according to either of these directions, but in a curve that will partake of both. And this curve will differ according to the nature and quantity of the forces that concurred to produce it.

as for instance, in many cases it will be such a curve as ends where it begun, or recurs into itself; that is, makes up a circle, like this ball; or an ellipsis, or oval, like this egg, which shall be further explained in our next course of Lectures.

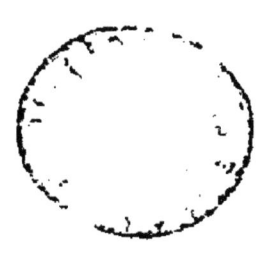

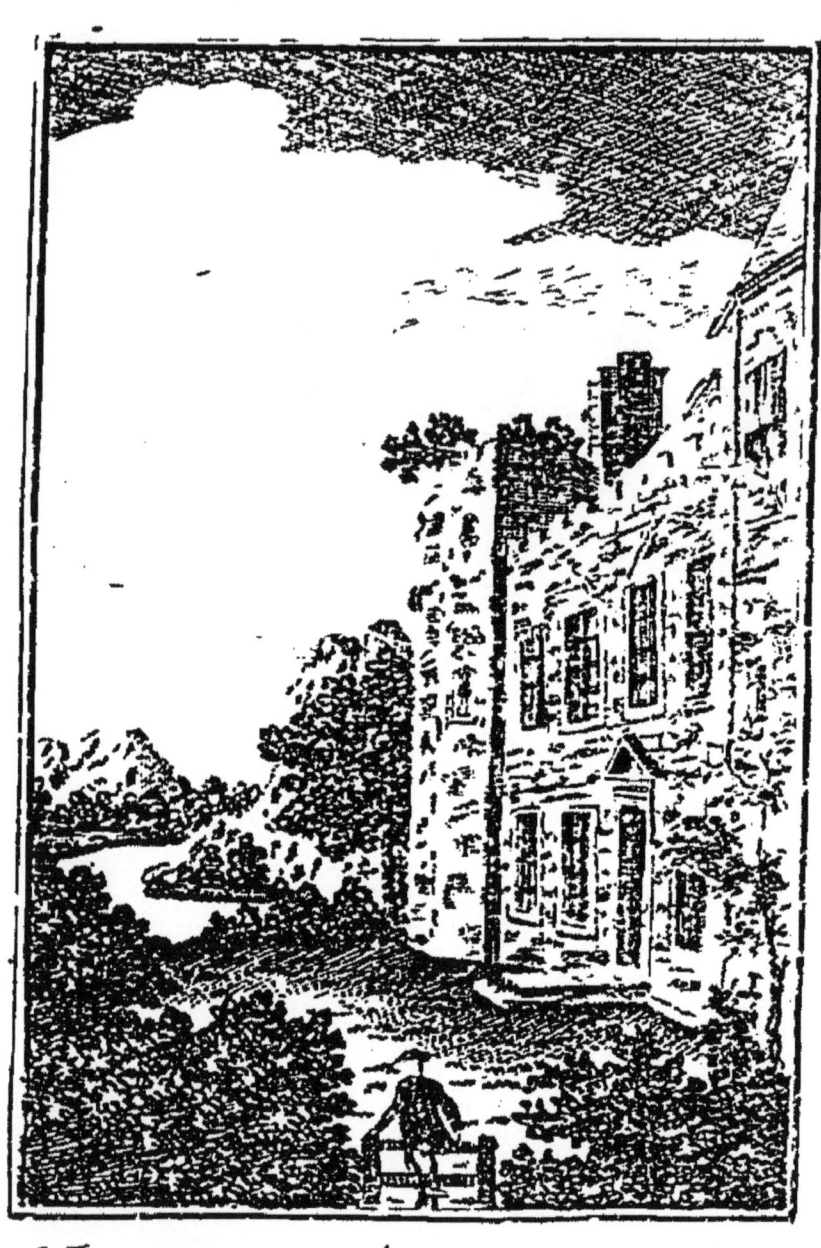

The Marquis of Bute's Observatory

LECTURE II.

Of the UNIVERSE, *and particularly of the* SOLAR SYSTEM.

THE laſt Lecture was read at the Marquis of *Setſtar's*, who was ſo well pleaſed at theſe young gentlemen's meeting thus to improve themſelves, that he ordered them to be elegantly treated with tarts, ſweetmeats, ſyllabubs, and ſuch other dainties as his Lordſhip thought were moſt proper for youth: and I muſt obſerve, that the Marchioneſs did them the honour of her company, and was particularly pleaſed with the converſation of Maſter *Teleſcope*. As it was a moonlight night, her Ladyſhip, after ſupper, led them to the top of a tower, where his Lordſhip has an obſervatory, furniſhed with all the inſtruments neceſſary for aſtronomical and philoſophical obſervations; and the place itſelf is the beſt that can be conceived for enquiries of this kind, and for meditation. To ſee an extenſive horizon thus ſhaded by the brow of night, and at intervals brightened up by the borrowed light of the moon dancing among the clouds,

clouds, was to me inexpressibly pleasing. Nothing was heard but a gentle breeze whispering the top of the battlements; the dying murmurs of a distant cascade; the malancholy hootings of the bird of night, who kept watch in an ivy tower near us; the mansion clock, that recorded the time; and old Echo, who repeated the hours from the side of a rock, where she has secluded herself ever since the deluge. Night, the nurse of Nature, hushed all things else to silence.——But silence was soon broke by our Philosopher, who thus began his Lecture.

Look round, my dear friends, says he, you see the earth seems to be bounded at an equal distance from us every way, where it appears to meet the sky, that forms this beautiful arch or concave over our heads. Now that distant round where we loose sight of the earth, is called the horizon, and when the sun, moon, and stars emerge from beneath and come into our sight, we say they are risen, or got above the horizon. For all this glorious canopy bespangled with lights, that bedeck the sky and illuminate the earth, as the *Sun*, the *Fixed Stars*, the *Comets* and *Planets*, (to which last our *Earth* and the *Moon* belong) have a 1

apparent

apparent motion, as may be perceived by the naked eye; though in fact none move but the planets and comets, as will be proved hereafter.

But besides the stars which we see, there are others not discernible by the naked eye, some of which are fixed stars, and some are bodies moving about the most distant planets, which were invisible and unknown to us before the discovery of prospective glasses.——Pray hand me the reflecting telescope.——Here it is.

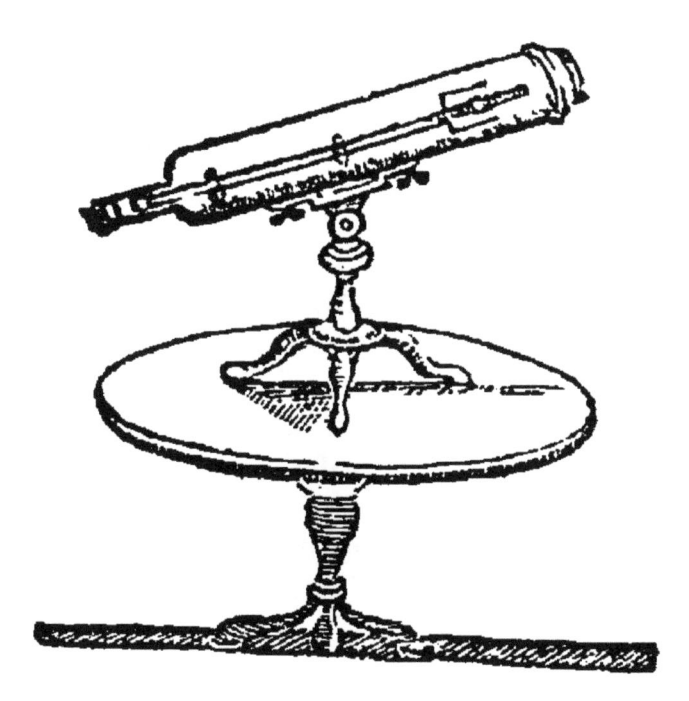

And the refracting telescope, if you please. ——Oh, here it is also.

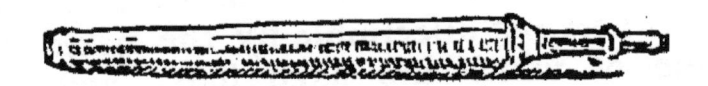

If you use the reflecting telescope, you must turn this screw on the side of it till you can see the object you want to examine in the most perfect manner; and if you use the refracting telescope, you must move backwards or forwards this small part, till you have adjusted it to your sight. Then look at that part of the heavens where I have pointed them, or indeed any other part, and you will perceive more stars than you saw before with your eye alone. These are fixed stars, and are called fixed, because they always keep the same distance one from another, and the same distance from the sun, which is supposed to be also fixed: and were he placed at the immense distance they are at, would probably appear no bigger than one of them. Hence some Philosophers have concluded, and I think not without reason, that every fixed star is
a sun

a sun that has a system of planets revolving round it, like our solar system. And if so, how immensely great, how wonderfully glorious, is the structure of this universe, which contains many thousand worlds, large as ours suspended in æther, rolling like the earth round their several suns, and filled with animals, plants, and minerals, all perhaps different from ours, but all intended to magnify the Almighty Architect; *who weighed the mountains in his golden scales, who measured the ocean in the hollow of his hand, who drew out the heavens as a curtain, who maketh the clouds his chariot, and walketh upon the wings of the wind.*

The fervour and air of piety, with which he delivered this, silenced all his companions, and gave infinite satisfaction to the Marchioness. Master *Wilson*, who had before been very impertinent, began now to consider himself as a fool in comparison of our Philosopher; and as Master *Telescope* had mentioned the solar system, he begged that he would explain it to him.

That I will with pleasure, replied the Philosopher; but first let me observe to you, that of these heavenly bodies some are *luminous*, and lend us their own light, as doth the *Sun* and *Fixed Stars*; while others are *opaque*, and have no light of their own to give us, but reflect to us a part of the light they receive from the sun. This is particularly the case with respect to the planets and comets of our solar system, which all give us a portion of the light they have received, and we in return reflect to them a portion of ours; for I make no doubt, but those who inhabit the moon have as much of the sun's light reflected to them from the earth, as we have reflected to us from the moon.

The inhabitants of the moon! says Master *Lovelace*, with some emotion, Whither will you lead me? What, are the stories that have been told of the Man in the Moon then true?

I don't know what stories you have heard, replied the Philosopher; but it is no extravagant conjecture to suppose, that the moon is inhabited as well as the earth; though what sort of inhabitants they are, we on the earth are unable to discover. As to my part, I am lost in this boundless abyss. It appears to me that the sun, which gives life to the world, is only a beam of the glory of God; and the air

which

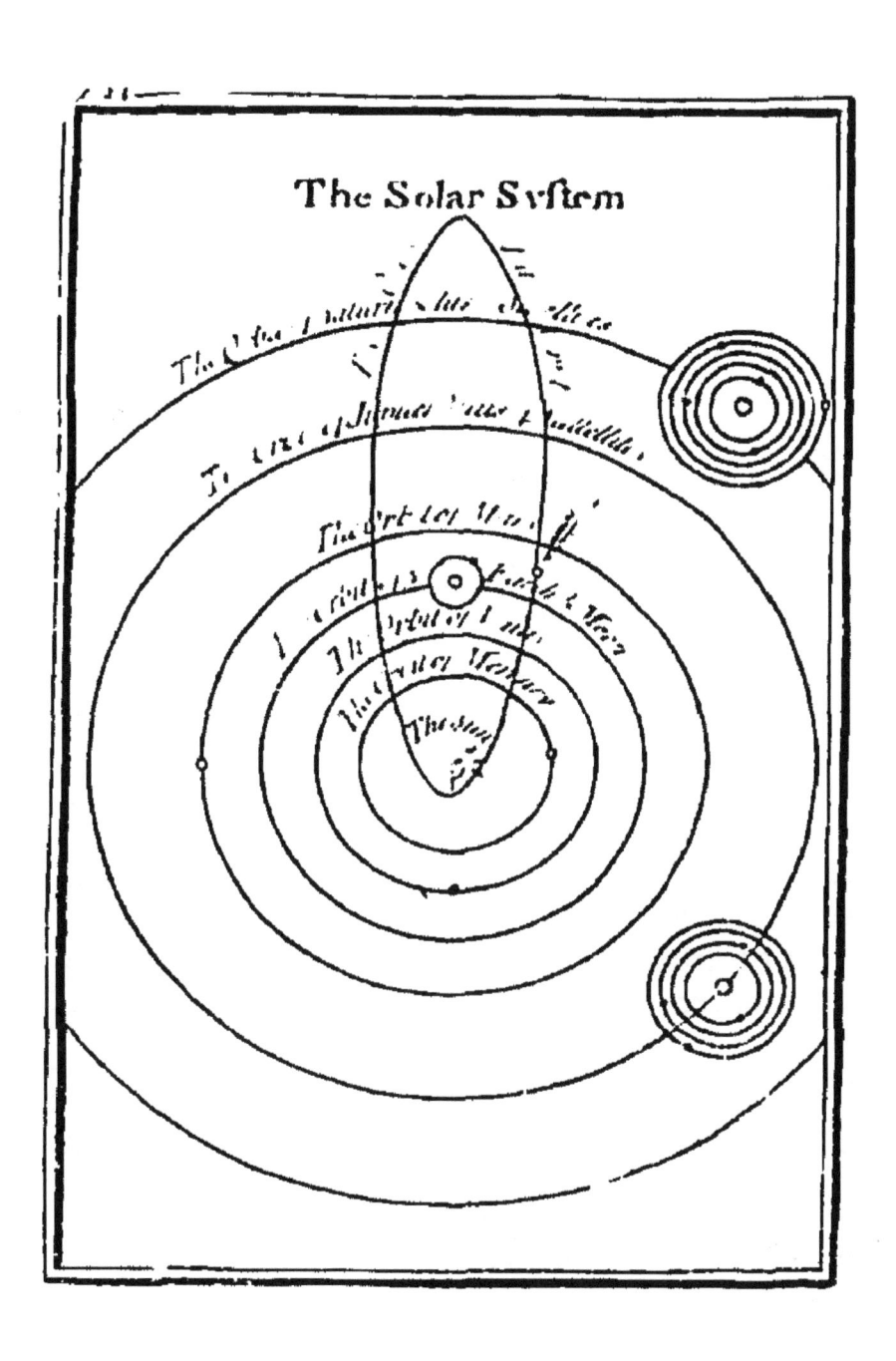

The Solar System

which supports that life, is, as it were, the breath of his nostrils.

Do thou, O God, support me while I gaze with astonishment at thy wonderful productions; since it is not idle impertinent curiosity that leads me to this enquiry, but a fervent desire to see only the skirts of thy glory, that I may magnify thy power and thy mercy to mankind.

Of the Solar System.

Our Solar System contains the sun in the centre, and the planets and comets moving about it ——— Pray look at the figure on the other side, where I have drawn the sun, and the planets in their several orbits or circles, with their respective distances from the sun, and from each other; together with the orbit of a comet.

The planets, as I have already observed, are bodies that appear like stars, but are not luminous; that is, they have no light in themselves, though they give us light, for they shine by reflecting the light of the sun. Of these there are two kinds, the one called *primary*, and the other *secondary* planets.

There are six *primary* planets, and these are *Mercury, Venus, the Earth, Mars, Ju-*
piter,

piter, and *Saturn*; all which move round the sun, as you may see in the figure before you, whereas the secondary planets move round other planets. The *Moon*, you know, (which is one of the *secondary* planets) moves round the *Earth*; four Moons, or *Satellites* as they are frequently called, move round *Jupiter*, and five round *Saturn*. And thus has the Almighty provided light for those regions that lie at such an immense distance from the sun.

The amazing distance, which each planet is at from the sun, may be seen by the time which each takes in its periodical revolution.

Mercury	⎫ revolves ⎧	83 days.
Venus	⎪ about the ⎪	225 days.
The Earth	⎬ Sun in the ⎨	365 d. 5 h. 49 m.
Mars	⎪ space of ⎪	1 year 322 days.
Jupiter	⎭ ⎩	11 years 319 days.
Saturn		29 years 138 days.

These move round about the Sun from west to east in the time above-mentioned. They are always to be found among the stars of those constellations that compose the twelve signs of the Zodiac; and in their progress do not describe a perfect circle, but an orbit a little inclining to an oval:
the

the reason whereof I shall give you in a future Lecture.

The comets move about the sun in a long slender oval of an amazing extent; one of the focus's being near the centre of the sun, and the shortest of the other far beyond the sphere of *Saturn*; so that the periodical revolutions of any are not performed in less than 70 or 80 years. See the *Plate*.

But let us quit these bodies, of which we know so little, and speak of our old companion the moon, with whom we ought to be better acquainted; since she not only lights us home in the night, but lends her aid to get our ships out of the docks, and to bring in and carry out our merchandize; for without the assistance of Lady *Luna* you would have no tides: but more of this hereafter.—A little more now, if you please, says *Tom Wilson*. What then, does the moon pour down water to occasion the tides? I am at a loss to understand you. No, replied our Philosopher, the moon does not pour down water to occasion the tides; that were impossible. but she, by attracting the waters of the sea, raises them higher, and that is the reason why the tides are always governed by the moon

The moon moves round the earth in the same manner as the earth does round the sun, and performs her synodical motion, as it is called, in 29 days, 12 hours, and 44 minutes, though the periodical is 27 days, 7 hours, and 43 minutes. By this motion of the moon are occasioned the eclipses of the sun and moon, and the different appearances, aspects, or phases she at different times puts on: for when the earth is so situated between the sun and the moon, that we see all her enlightened parts, it is *full Moon*; when the moon is so situated between the sun and the earth, that her enlightened parts are hid or turned from us, it is *new Moon*, and when her situation is such, that only a portion of her enlightened part is hid from us, we see a *horned Moon*, a *half Moon*, or a *gibbous Moon*, according to the quantity of the enlightened part we can perceive.

The total or longest *Eclipse of the Moon* happens when the earth is directly between the sun and the moon, and prevents the light of the sun from falling upon and being reflected by the moon, as I'll shew you. We will supose this orange to be the sun, this cricket-ball the earth, and this up the moon, now if you place them in

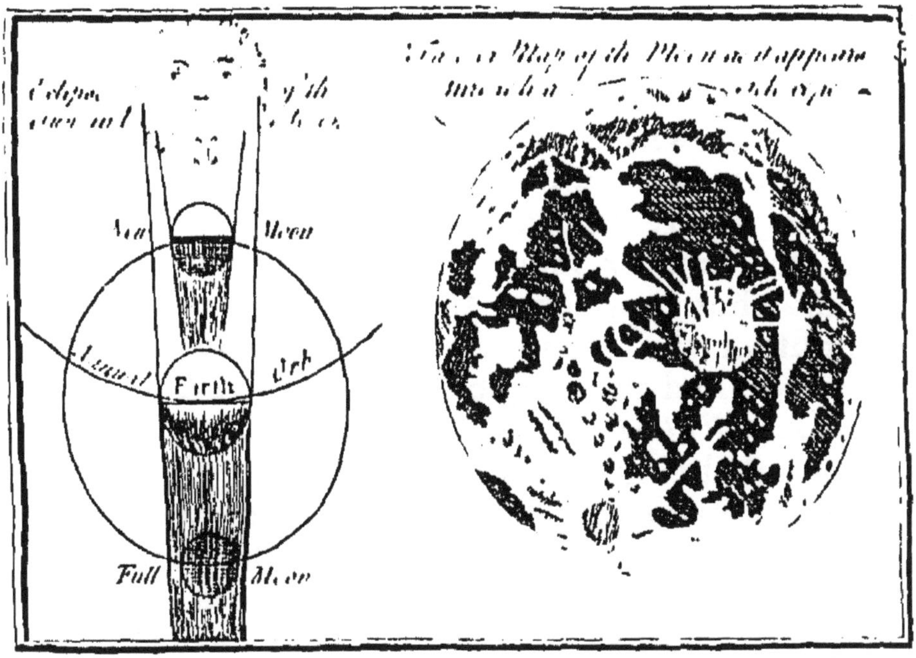

New
Moon
Earth
Full
Moon

a straight line, with the ball in the middle, and then put your eye to the top, you'll find that the ball will entirely hide the orange from your view, and would prevent the rays of light (which always proceed in right lines) from falling upon it, whence would ensue a *total* eclipse. But move the top, which represents the moon, a little on either side, and with your eye placed as before, you will perceive a part of the orange, which will be now in such a position, that a straight line may be drawn from a part of the orange or sun, to a part of the top or moon, without touching the ball that represents the earth, and in this position the moon would be partly illuminated, and the eclipse be only *partial.*

An *Eclipse of the Sun* is occasioned by the moon's being betwixt the sun and the earth, and preventing the light of the sun from coming to that part of the earth which we inhabit —If the moon hides from us the whole body of the sun, it is a *total* eclipse; but if the whole be not hid, it is a *partial* one. An *Eclipse* of the *Sun* never happens but at a *new* Moon, nor one of the *Moon* but when she is at the *full.*

The Moon, as to matter and form, appears not much unlike our earth, as you may

may perceive by this Map. The bright parts are supposed to be the high illuminated tracts of land, as *mountains*, *islands*, &c. and the dark parts, it is imagined, are the *seas*, *lakes*, and *vales*, which reflect but little light. But of this there is no certainty.

The *Earth*, by its revolution about the sun in 365 days, 5 hours, and 49 minutes, measures out that space of time which we call a *Year*, and the line described by the earth in this annual revolution about the sun is called the *Ecliptic*. To give you a perfect idea of this and other circles necessary to be known, I have on the opposite side presented you with the figure of a sphere.

The annual motion of the earth round the sun is from west to east, or to speak more philosophically, it is according to the order of the signs of the *Zodiac*; which we shall hereafter explain.

But besides this annual motion or revolution about the sun in the line of the *Ecliptic*, the earth turns round upon its own axis in about 24 hours; so that it hath two motions at one and the same time.

The Marchioness, whose curiosity had kept her there during the Lecture, desired to have this explained. That shall be done, Madam,

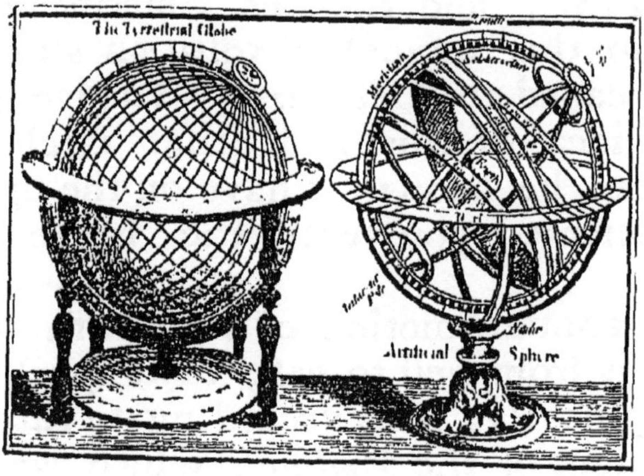
The Terrestrial Globe
Nadir
Artificial Sphere

Madam, in a minute, says the little Philosopher, and I can never have a better opportunity; for I see the Duke of *Galaxy* is coming to make your Ladyship a visit. His coach is just entering the iron gates, and will presently wheel round the circle, or rather oval, before the portico. Pray, Madam, fix your eyes on one of the wheels, which you may do as it is moon-light, and you will perceive it turn round upon its own axis, at the same time that it runs round the circle before the house. This double motion of the wheel very fitly represents the two motions of the earth, which have heretofore been explained by the motion of a bowl on a bowling-green; but I believe your Ladyship will think the instance or example before us is better. It is hard to reason from similitudes, because they generally fail in some part: all the members of a simile seldom correspond with the subject it is intended to illustrate; and, if I mistake not, that is the case with the bowl upon the green, which, though it aptly represents the earth's motion on its own axis, is far from representing its revolution about the sun, because the bias in the bowl will never induce it to form either a circle or an oval; for the figure it describes is

rather

rather a parabola, or that fort of figure which a long fifhing-rod forms, when it is bent by drawing a fifh out of the water.

Your Ladyfhip knows perfectly that the earth turning on its own axis makes the difference of the day and night: you will therefore give me leave, Madam, to addrefs my difcourfe to thefe young gentlemen and ladies, who may be ignorant of this branch of Philofophy.

That the turning of the earth on its own axis makes the difference of *day* and *night* is moft certain; for in thofe parts of the earth which are turned towards the fun it will be *day*, and of confequence it muft be *night* in thofe which are turned from it.

But the length of *days* and *nights*, and the variations of the *feafons*, are occafioned by the annual revolution of the earth about the fun in the *Ecliptic*; for as the earth in this courfe keeps its axis equally inclined every where to the plane of the Ecliptic and parallel to itfelf, and as the plane of the Ecliptic inclines 23 degrees and a half towards the Equator, the earth in this direction has fometimes one of its poles neareft the fun, and fometimes the other. Hence heat and cold, fummer and winter,
and

and length of days and nights. Yet notwithstanding these effects of the sun, which gives us light and heat, his distance from us is so great, that a cannon-ball would be twenty-five years coming from thence to the earth, even if it flew with the same velocity as it does when it is first discharged from the mouth of a cannon.

Here they were all amazed, and Lady *Caroline* said this doctrine could not be true; for if the sun were at that immense distance, his light could not reach us every morning, in the manner it does.——I beg your pardon, Madam, replied the Philosopher; your Ladyship's mistake arises from your not knowing, or at least not considering, the amazing velocity of light which flies after the rate of 200,000 miles in a *second* of time; so that notwithstanding a cannon-ball wou'd be 25 years in coming from the sun, the light finds its way to us in about eight minutes. But if you are so surprized at the sun's distance, Madam, what think you of that of the fixed stars, which are so far remote from us, that a cannon ball, flying with the same velocity as when first discharged, would be 700,000 years in coming to the earth? Yet many of these stars are seen, and even without the use of telescopes.

There are other things observable in our Solar System, which if attended to will excite our admiration: such as the dark spots which are seen on the *Sun's* surface, and which often change their *place, number,* and *magnitude.* Such also is the amazing Ring which encompasses the body of the planet *Saturn* at the distance of 21,000 miles; and such are the belts that gird the body of *Jupiter:* concerning all which there are various conjectures; but conjectures in Philosophy are rarely to be admitted.

LECTURE III.

Of the AIR, ATMOSPHERE, and METEORS.

WHAT was said by the Marchioness and Lady *Caroline* in favour of Master *Telescope* excited the Duke of *Galaxy's* curiosity to see him, and the next morning he came into the Observatory just as the Lecture began. The presence of so great

great a personage as the Duke put our young gentlemen into some confusion, and several of them offered to go away; which the Duke observing, stepped into the next room, and Master *Telescope* took this opportunity to correct their folly.

Gentlemen, says he, I am amazed at your meanness and ill manners. What, because the Duke does you the honour of a visit, will you run away from him? There is nothing betrays a mean spirit and low education so much as this ridiculous awe and dread which some people shew in the company of their superiors; and besides it is troublesome; for the uneasiness one person is in communicates itself to the rest of the company, and abridges them of a portion of their pleasure. The easier you appear in the company of the great, the more polite you will be esteemed. None but a clown hangs down his head, and hides his face; for a gentleman always looks in the face of his superior when he talks to him, and behaves with openness and freedom. As to my part, I venerate his Grace; but then it is for his great worthiness of character, which has engaged my affection, and inclines me to wish for his company, not to avoid it. *Civility we owe*

34 *Of the* AIR, ATMOSPHERE, &c.

owe to every one, and *Respect* is due to the Great: it is claimed, and it is given, in consequence of their superior birth and fortune, but that is all; for our affection is only to be obtained by worthiness of character. Birth and fortune are merely accidental, and may happen to be the portion of a man without merit, but the man of genius and virtue is ennobled as it were by himself, and is honoured not so much for his grandfather's greatness as his own. This reproof had its proper effect, for they all sat down, and his Grace being returned, with Lady *Caroline*, our Philosopher began his Lecture on the nature and properties of the *Air*, *Atmosphere*, and *Meteors* contained therein.

We have already considered the earth as a planet, says he, and observed its diurnal and annual motion, we are now to speak of the materials of which it is composed, and of the Atmosphere, and the Meteors that surround and attend it.

In order to explain these effectually, says the Duke, you should, I think, Sir, begin with an account of the first principles or four Elements, which are *Fire*, *Air*, *Earth*, and *Water*, and then shew how they effect each other, and by their mutual aid give
motion,

motion, life and spirit to all things, for without fire the water would assume a different form, and become solid ice; without water the fire would scorch up the earth, and destroy both animals and plants; without air, the fire perhaps would be unable to execute its office, nor without air could the water, though exhaled by the sun into clouds, be distributed over the earth for the nourishment of plants and animals. Nor is the earth inactive, but lends her aid to the other elements. She filters, or strains and purifies, the salt-water which runs from the sea, and makes it fresh and fit for the use of animals and plants; and, by reflecting the sun's beams, occasions that warmth which nourishes all things on her surface; but which would be very inconsiderable and scarcely felt, if a man was placed on the highest mountain, above the common level of the earth, and in such a situation as to be deprived of her reflection.

All this, my Lord Duke, I have considered, replied the Philosopher, and had thoughts of carrying it farther, and shewing how those elements pervade and are become indeed constituent parts of the same body, for *Fire*, *Air*, *Earth*, and *Water*, are to be drawn even from a dry stick of wood. That two sticks rubbed violently together will produce fire is very well known; for coach or waggon wheels frequently take fire when not properly clouted with iron, and supplied with grease. And if pieces of wood, seemingly dry, be put into a glass retort over a furnace, you'll obtain both air and water, and then if you burn the wood to ashes, and wash out the salts with water, as the good women do when they make lye, the remaining part will be pure earth: And thus we can at any time draw the four elements out of a stick of wood. But as these speculations are above the comprehension of some of the young gentlemen whom I have the honour to instruct, I shall defer the consideration of such minute and abstruse matters till another opportunity. Science is to be taught as we teach children the use of their legs; they are at first shewn how to stand alone, after this they are taught to walk with safety, and then suffered to run as fast as they please. And I beg your Grace will permit me to pursue this method in the course of my Lectures. The Duke gave his assent with a nod, and our Philosopher thus proceeded.

The

Of the AIR, ATMOSPHERE, &c.

The air is a light, thin, elastic or springy body, which may be felt but not seen; it is fluid, and runs in a current like water, (as you may perceive by opening the window) but it cannot, like water, be congealed into ice; and the Atmosphere is that great body or shell of air which surrounds the earth, and which reaches many miles above its surface, as is known by considering the elasticity or springiness of the air and its weight together; for a column of air is of equal weight to a column of quicksilver, of between 29 and 30 inches high; now quicksilver being near fourteen times heavier than water, if the air was as heavy as water, the Atmosphere would be about fourteen times higher than the column of quicksilver, or about 34 feet, but the air is near 1000 times lighter than water; therefore the Atmosphere must be many miles high, even at this rate of computing: And when with this you consider the elasticity of the air, which, when the pressure of the incumbent Atmosphere is taken off, will dilate itself so as to fill more than 150 times the space it occupied before, you will perceive that the height of the Atmosphere must be very great.

38 Of the Air, Atmosphere, &c.

For as the air is a springy body, that part next the earth must be more dense than the upper part, as being pressed down by the air above it. Look at that hay-stack yonder, which the groom is cutting, and you'll perceive that the hay at the bottom is much closer and harder to cut than that at the top, because it has been pressed into less space than it otherwise would have occupied, by the other hay above it, and had not the whole stack been trodden and pressed down by the man who made it, the difference would have been still more considerable.

The air, however, even near the earth, is not always in the same state. It is sometimes rarified, and becomes lighter than at other times, as appears by the quicksilver's falling in the Barometer, and the rain's descending on the earth, for it is the dense state or weight of the air, which raises the quicksilver in the Barometer, and the water in the pump, and prevents the clouds from falling down in rain.

The elastic principle in the air, which renders it so capable of being rarified and condensed, has been productive of the most wonderful effects. But before you proceed farther,

farther, says Lady *Caroline*, pray do me the favour, Sir, to convince me, by some experiment, that the air is endowed with this wonderful quality. That he cannot do, replied the Duke, without the use of proper instruments. Almost any thing will do, an't please your Grace, says the Philosopher.—Little Master's *Pop Gun* that lies in the window is sufficient for my purpose — Do me the honour to step this way, Lady *Caroline*. You see here is a pellet in the top of this tube, made of hemp or brown paper. With this piece of paper we will make another pellet, and put it into the other end. Now with the gun stick drive it forward. There you have forced the pellet some part of the way with ease, but it will be more difficult to get it farther, because the air, being compressed and made more dense or compact, will make more resistance; and when you have pressed it so close that its force overpowers the resistance which the pellet makes at the other end, that pellet will fly off with a bounce, and be thrown by the spring of the air to a considerable distance.—There see with what force it is thrown.

This you have taken little notice of, because it is a school boy's action, and is seen every day; for, indeed, we seldom trouble ourselves to reason about things that are so familiar, yet on this principle, my Lady, depends the force of a cannon; for it is not the gunpowder and fire that drives out the ball with such prodigious velocity; no, that force is occasioned by the fire's suddenly rarifying the air which was contained in the chamber or breech of the cannon, and that generated by the powder itself. As a proof of this, place the same ball in the same quantity of powder in an open vessel, and when fired you will scarce see it move. But there have been guns lately invented, called wind-guns, which abundantly prove what I have advanced, for they are charged only with concentrated or condensed air and with ball, yet are so contrived, that six or seven balls may be let off, one after the other, each of which would kill a buck or a doe at a very considerable distance.

You seem all amazed, and I don't wonder at it, since you have never yet considered the extraordinary properties of this element; and it must seem strange to you that the

the air, which is so necessary for life that without it we cannot breathe, should be tortured into an instrument of destruction. You will, however, be more surprised when I tell you that this is probably the cause of earthquakes, and that the noble city of *Lisbon* was lately destroyed by a sudden rarifaction of the air contained in some of the caverns of the earth, and perhaps under the sea. *Tom Wilson* gave a leer of impertinence, but was ashamed to shew his folly before such good company. All the rest stared at each other without speaking a word, except Lady *Caroline*, who protested she could not believe what he had said about earthquakes; for, says she, I remember to have read in the News papers, that the flames burst out of the ground. That might be, my Lady, says the little Philosopher, for there could be no such sudden rarifaction of the air without fire. Fire, therefore, did contribute towards the earthquake, and fire might burn down a mountain composed of combustibles; but fire could never blow one up. No, my Lady, that effect is the sole property of the air. This dispute would, in all probability, have taken up much time, but his Grace

put

put an end to the controversy, by declaring it was true Philosophy.

In this property of being rarified and condensed, the air differs amazingly from water, which, though composed of such small particles as not to be distinguished or seen separately with a microscope, and notwithstanding its readiness to rise or be evaporated with heat, and to be separated with a touch, cannot, when confined, be at all concentrated or brought into a less compass. This experiment was once tried, by filling a golden globe full of water, then closing it up, and placing it in a screw press, which was pulled down with great force. In this situation it remained till the water sweated through the pores of the gold, and till that happened it would never give way.

Air is the medium which diffuses light to the world; for if there was no Atmosphere to refract the sun's rays round the globe, it would be almost as dark in the day time as in the night, and the *Sun*, *Moon*, and *Stars*, would only be visible. It is also the medium of sounds, which are conveyed by the tremulous motion of the air when agitated by any noise. Let me throw this peach stone into the moat, and
you

Of the Air, Atmosphere, &c.   43

you will perceive circles of small waves diffuse themselves by degrees to a great distance round it. Now as the air is fluid as well as the water, we may conclude that sound is conveyed somewhat in this manner, though as that is nearly a thousand times lighter than water, sounds are propagated at an amazing rate, some say after the rate of 1142 feet in a second of time, but however that be, we may rest assured, that sound is conveyed in this manner. Only throw up the sash, and halloo, and the echo, which I spoke of in the beginning of the second Lecture, will return you the sound; that is, the waves or pulses of air, which are put in motion by the noise you make, will strike against the rocks, and return to you again, for echo is nothing but the *reverberation* of sound. And that there can be no sound conveyed without air is proved by experiment; for a bell, struck in an exhausted receiver in an air pump, cannot be heard, that is, it has little or no sound.

Without air there would be no merchandize, for your ships could not sail to foreign climates; and without air the birds could not fly, since they would have nothing

thing to support them, and their wings would be useless; for we know, that a feather falls with as much velocity as a guinea in an exhausted receiver. But above all, air is the principle which preserves life, both in plants and animals; there is no breathing without air, and you know, when our breath is stopt, we die. This is one of those truths that are called self evident, because it is universally known, and needs no confirmation; but, if demonstration be thought necessary, you may have it in a minute, by putting some living creature into the air pump, but it is cruel to torture a poor animal: So said Lady *Caroline*, and violently opposed this experiment's being tried; but as all the rest were for it, the Duke was willing to gratify their curiosity, and therefore told our Philosopher, that he might try the experiment with a rat, which they had caught in a trap, and if he survived it, give him his life for the pain they had put him to. This creature was accordingly put into the receiver, and, when the air was partly exhausted, he appeared in great agony, and convulsed; and more air being pumped out, he fell on his side for
dead;

The Air-Gun

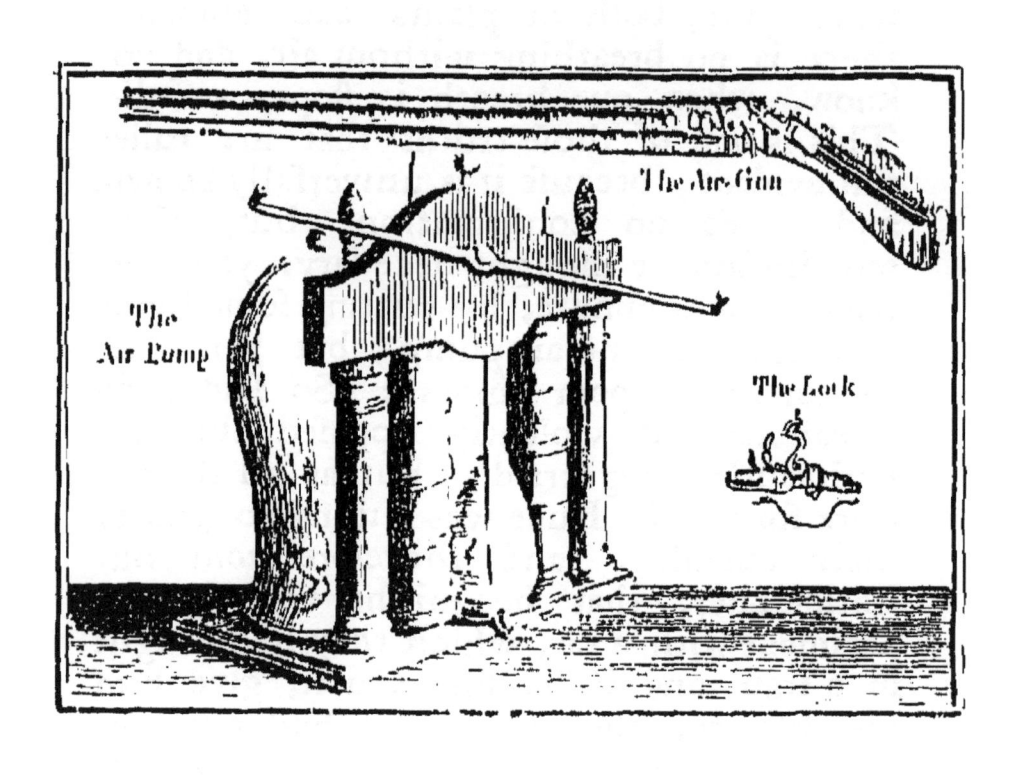

The Air Pump

The Lock

dead; but fresh air being immediately admitted, it rushed into his lungs, which put them in motion again, and he recovered. The manner of the animal's recovery puts me in mind, says the Philosopher, of an accident which I once saw, and which I would have you all remember, for it may be of service to mankind.

Some time ago I was bathing, with several of my school fellows, in a river by the road side. Master *Curtis*, who was an obstinate silly boy, would dastard the rest, as he called it; that is, he would foolishly exceed them in running into dangers and difficulties, and with this view, though he could swim no more than a stone, he plunged into a part of the river, which we told him was greatly above his depth, where he rose and struggled to get out, but could not. We were all, you must imagine, in the utmost distress, and unable to assist him, for none of us could swim. At this instant came by some Gentlemen on horseback, who immediately dismounted, and got him out, but not till after he had sunk the third time. He was brought to the shore without figns of life, and blooded without any effect; when one of the Gentlemen, who, I have since heard, was a great Philosopher, advised them to blow some air down his throat; this was done, and the elasticity of the air put his lungs in motion, as I imagine, for a pulsation immediately ensued, he recovered almost as soon as this animal. Now, from what I heard that Gentleman say, and from the instance before us, there is reason to believe, that the lives of many might be saved, who are supposed drowned, if this method was put in practice of conveying air to the lungs, for you are to consider; that unless the lungs are in motion, there can be no circulation; and it was for want of air that their motion ceased in the water. Pray, Gentlemen, let this be remembered, for it is a matter of great importance.

We are to observe, Gentlemen, that air which has passed through fire, or is become foul, or stagnated, and has lost its spring, is unfit for respiration. It was the want of fresh air, or in other words, the being obliged to breathe air that was foul, and had lost its spring, or elastic force, that

killed

killed so many of our poor countrymen in the black hole at *Calcutta* in the *East-Indies*, as you have seen by the newspapers; and this breathing of foul air in inflammatory, putrid, and eruptive disorders, such, for instance, as the small-pox, and some fevers, has destroyed more than can be imagined. If therefore you should be seized with any of these disorders advise the people about you to make use of their common sense, and not, because a man is ill, deprive him of that vital principle the air, without which he could not live, even in a state of health. Never suffer your curtains to be drawn close, or exclude the fresh air even when you sleep.

I am greatly mistaken, says Lady *Caroline*, if the air we are now in has not lost its spring; for I breathe with difficulty. Was that the case, Madam, replied the little Philosopher, you would not be able to breathe at all; but if your Ladyship finds the air so disposed, you should make use of the instrument that lies by you, which, by putting the air in motion, will in part recover its spring. What instrument, Sir? says the Lady Your fan, Madam,

Madam, returned the Philosopher. Every fan is a philosophical instrument, and was originally contrived, we may suppose, for the purpose above mentioned.

A bird dying in an air-pump will be in some measure recovered by the convulsive fluttering of his own wings, because that motion alters the state of the air remaining in the receiver, and for a time renders it fit for respiration.

Motion is the only preservative for air and water; both of which become unwholsome if kept long in a state of rest; and both may be recovered and made salutary by being again put into motion.

If foul and stagnated air has such dire effects, how much are we obliged to the learned and ingenious Dr. *Hales* for discovering the *Ventilator*, an instrument which, in a little time, discharges the foul air from ships, prisons, and other close places, and supplies them with that which is fresh?

The air, by some Philosophers, has been esteemed an universal *menstruum*, because, say they, it dissolves all bodies in time, and reduces their substances to a new form; as iron into rust, copper into verdigrease, *&c.* but this, I am inclined to think, is not so much owing to the air as to certain saline

or

Of the AIR, ATMOSPHERE, &c. 49

or acid particles, which the air extracts from those bodies, and which afterwards cleave to other bodies, with which they have a closer affinity, than with the air itself. But this I shall endeavour to explain in a future work.

We are now to speak of the Wind, which is only a stream or current of air, as a river is of water, and is occasioned by heat, eruptions of vapours, condensations, rarifactions, the pressure of clouds, the fall of rains, or some other accident that disturbs the equilibrium of the air, for Nature abhors a vacuum, and for that reason, when the air is extremely rarified in one part, that which is more dense will immediately rush in to supply the vacant places, and preserve the equilibrium, as is the case with water and other fluid substances. Only raise a vessel of water suddenly out of a cistern, and see with what speed the other water will rush in, to fill up the space and preserve it's level. And these rarifactions in the air may happen near the earth, or much above it, and is the reason why clouds fly in contrary directions. This occasioned the loss of the great *Kite*, which we were a whole fortnight in making, for, though there was scarcely wind in the Park sufficient to raise it, yet when lifted extremely high by the air, it was seized by a current of wind and torn in pieces.

Winds are violent, or gentle, in proportion to the rarifaction or disturbance there has been in the atmosphere. A violent wind, in a great storm, flies after the rate of 50 or 60 miles in an hour, and is often so dense, or strong, as to bear down trees, houses, and even churches before it. What the sailors call a brisk wind flies after the rate of about 15 miles an hour, and is of great use in cooling the air, and cleansing it from poisonous and pestilential exhalations.

The winds have various qualities, they are generally hot or cold, according to the quarter from whence they blow. I remember, some years ago we had a South-West wind in *February*, which blew so long from that quarter, that it brought us the very air of *Lisbon*, and it was as hot as in summer. Winds from the North and North-East, which come off large tracts of land, are generally cold. Some winds moisten and dissolve, others dry and thicken: some raise rain, and others disperse it: some winds blow constantly from one quarter,

ter, and are therefore called the *general Trade Winds*. These are met with on each side of the *Equator* in the *Atlantic, Ethiopic, and Pacific Oceans*, between the Tropicks, and to near 24 degrees of latitude; and are occasioned by the Sun in his rotation round his axis, agitating the æther, or by the rarifaction of the air by the solar rays, and the denser air continually pouring in from the distant parts of each hemisphere to maintain the equilibrium. Some winds, again, blow constantly one way for one half, or one quarter of the year, and then blow the contrary way. These are met with in the *East Indian Seas*, and are called *Monsoons*, or periodical Trade Winds. But as these subjects are abstruse and difficult, and afford little entertainment, we shall defer an explanation of them till our next course of Lectures, and endeavour to give you some account of the Meteors that attend the air.

We have already observed, that, besides pure air, the atmosphere contains minute particles of different sorts, which are continually arising in streams from the earth and waters, and are suspended and kept floating in the air.

The

The most considerable of these are the small particles of water, which are so separated as to be lighter than air, and are raised by the Sun's heat, or lifted up by the wind from the sea, rivers, lakes, and marshy or moist parts of the earth, and which descend again in *Dews, Rain, Hail,* and *Snow.*

When these small particles are, by a rarified state of the air, suffered to unite many of them together, and descend so as to render the hemisphere more opaque, and by its humidity to moisten bodies on the earth, it is called a *Mist.* And, on the contrary, those particles of water that arise after a hot day from rivers, lakes, and marshy places, and by filling the air moisten objects and render them less visible, are called *Fogs.*

Clouds are the greatest and most beneficial of all the *meteors*, for they are borne about on the wings of the wind, and, as the Psalmist observes, *Distribute fatness to the earth.* Clouds contain very small particles of water, which are raised a considerable distance above the surface of the earth, for a cloud is nothing but a mist flying high in the air, as a mist is nothing but a cloud here below.

That these vapours are raised in the air,
in

in the manner above-mentioned, may be readily conceived, for it is an action that is seen every day in common distillations, but how these invisible particles, which float in the air, are collected into clouds in order to bring the water back again, is not so easy to determine. Perhaps, says the Marchioness, who had just before entered the room, it may be occasioned by the winds driving the clouds together and uniting the particles, which may by that means become specifically heavier than the air, and therefore fall down. There is reason, my Lady, in what you say, replied the Philosopher, but I would wish to know how these clouds are sometimes all of a sudden collected It frequently happens, Madam, that you go abroad when the sky is so serene and clear, that not a cloud is to be seen, and before your Ladyship has taken a turn round the *Park*, you shall see clouds gather round, and all the hemisphere overcast, and the drops begin to fall. How happens this? There were no clouds for the winds to drive against each other, nor could the aqueous vapours arise from the earth, and descend at the same instant of time. Whence then could they come?

I am

I am afraid, Madam, says the Duke, this young Gentleman has shaken your Ladyship's Philosophy; for the question he has put is not to be answered without some knowledge of Chemistry, which is, I think, too little studied in this kingdom. I am not uneasy about it, my Lord Duke, says the Marchioness, he is the Lecturer, and let him account for it if he can.—I shall get little honour by solving this question, says the Philosopher, since his Grace has pointed out the only method, by which it can be done, that is to say, by Chemistry, for that action of bodies which the Chemists call *precipitation*, will answer it in all respects; but the explanation of it is a task so difficult, that I must defer it till another opportunity. Some idea, however, I will endeavour to give these young Gentlemen of precipitation, if your Ladyship will favour me with that tincture of bark which I saw in your hand this morning. The bark, Gentlemen, at least the resinous part of the bark, is here suspended in the spirits of wine; and so suspended, that you see it is perfectly bright. Now, in order to precipitate this bark, I must find out a body which has a closer affinity or relation with the spirits of wine,
than

Of the Air, Atmosphere, &c.

than the bark has (for things inanimate have all their relations when chemically confidered,) that body is water, which when I add to the tincture, you will perceive it grow foul; for the spirits of wine will immediately let go the bark to lay hold of the water, which will occupy the space the bark before filled, and that will fall to the bottom. This perhaps may be the case in the atmosphere: some substance my be brought into the air, to which it is nearer allied than to the water, that it suspended before in such a pellucid manner, as not to be seen, but which water becomes obvious, when the air lets it go to embrace its nearer ally, and by uniting first into small drops, then into larger, becomes too heavy to be suspended by the air, and falls down in *rain*.

But all clouds are not composed of watery vapours only, they are sometimes impregnated with sulphureous and even saline particles, which are exhaled from the earth; for the Chemists will tell you by experience, that volatile bodies will volatilize some fixed bodies, and carry them off: And this happens to be the case here, as may be particularly seen in *Thunder* and *Lightning*, which is occasioned, we may suppose, by the

the sulphureous and nitrous particles taking fire, and bursting the cloud with a tremendous noise, which is proceeded by a flash of fire, much resembling that of lighted *gun-powder*, only more penetrating, which is owing, perhaps, to its extreme volatility.—But look, there is a cloud rising before us, which seems replete with that electrical matter, and may by and by discover, in a more sensible manner, those effects to you which I have been endeavouring to describe.

That there are some sort of nitrous particles, or a substance very much like it, raised in the air, is, I think, evident from that nourishment which rain (and particularly that rain which is attended with thunder) gives to vegetables, above common water, and from the quantities of nitre which have been found in heaps of earth that were exposed to the air, at the same time that it was kept from the rain.

Snow seems to be the small particles of water frozen in the air before they had united into drops, and *hail* seems to be drops of rain frozen in the fall From the regular figures which *snow* and *hail* put on in their descent, some have been inclined to think that they contain particles of salt
mixed

mixed with the water, and which occasioned them to shoot and unite in certain angles; but an experiment should, I think, be tried before this is admitted as true Philosophy, and it might be done by boiling the snow and hail over the fire, till it put on a pellicle or scum at the top, and then setting it in a cold place, for the salts to crystallize, or shoot to the bottom.

"I know nothing of Crystallizations, says Lady *Caroline*, nor shall I ever turn Chemist; therefore, good Sir, give us something more entertaining. Pray can you tell me what occasioned those terrible lights in the air which we had last week?"

The *Aurora Borealis*, or northern lights, says he, are occasioned, Madam, by certain *nitrous* and *sulphureous vapours*, which are thinly spread through the atmosphere above the clouds, where they ferment, and taking fire, the *explosion* of one portion kindles the next, and the flashes succeed one another, till all the vapour is set on fire, the streams whereof seem to converge towards the zenith of the spectator, or that point of the heavens which is immediately over his head.

At this instant, up started Master *Long*, and told her Ladyship, if she had done, he he would be glad to aſk a queſtion. Sir, ſays ſhe, with a ſmile, it was you made the compliment, I ſhould be glad to hear your queſtion, for, I dare ſay, it would be a ſenſible one. I wiſh you may find it ſo, replied he, but what I want to have an account of, is this ſame *Jack with-a-Lantern*, which ſo haunts my Lord Marquis's park; and t'other day led my friend *Tom Wilſon* into a large pond. Miſter *Wilſon*, you are to underſtand, had been at his uncle's, where he ſtaid rather too late, and therefore his uncle ordered the footman to light him home, but *Tom*, being a very courageous fellow, and a little obſtinate, would walk home alone, and in the dark but juſt as he came into the marſhy meadow, who ſhould he almoſt overtake but this ſame Gentleman, this *Jack-with a-Lantern*, whom he miſtook for Goody *Curtis*, the chairwoman, and thought ſhe was lighting herſelf home from work. *Tom* ran to overtake Dame *Curtis*, but Mr. *Jack-with his-Lantern* ſtill kept out of reach, and led my friend *Tom* out of the path, which he did not perceive till he had loſt himſelf, on which *Tom* ran, and *Jack* ran. *Tom* halloo'd, and *Jack* would not anſwer; at laſt

ſouſe

souse came *Tom* into *Duckweed Pond*, where he might have lain till this time, if Mr. *Goodall* had not heard him call out, as he was riding by, and ran to his assistance. This put all the company in good humour, and *Tom* had good nature and good sense enough to join them in the laugh, which being subsided, our Philosopher thus proceeded in his Lecture.

The *Ignis Fatuus*, *Jack with-a-Lantern*, or *Will-with-the-Wisp*, as it is frequently called, says he, is supposed to be only a *fat, unctuous,* and *sulphureous vapour*, which in the night appears lucid, and being driven about by the air near the earth's surface, is often mistaken for a light in a lantern, as my friend Master *Wilson* can testify. Vapours of this kind are in the night frequently kindled in the air, and some of them appear like falling stars, and are by ignorant people so called.

It may be here necessary to mention that beautiful phenomenon the Rainbow, since it has the appearance of a meteor, though, in reality, it is none; for the Rainbow is occasioned by the refraction or reflection of the sun's beams from the very small drops of a cloud or mist seen in a certain angle made by two lines, the one drawn from the sun, and the other from the eye of the spectator, to those small drops in the cloud which reflect the sun's beams. So that two persons, looking on a Rainbow at the same time, do not, in reality, see the same Rainbow.

There are other appearances in the atmosphere which ought to be taken notice of, and these are the halos, or circles, which sometimes seem to encompass the sun and moon, and are often of different colours. These always appear in a *rimy* or *frosty* season, and are therefore, we may suppose, occasioned by the refraction of light in the frozen particles in the air.

Here the Lecture would have ended, but a sudden clap of thunder brought on fresh matter for meditation; some of the company, and particularly the Ladies, endeavoured to avoid the lightning, but Master *Telescope*, after the second clap, threw up the sash, and assured the Ladies and Gentlemen there was no danger, for that the clouds were very high in the air. The danger in a thunder storm, says he, is in proportion to the violence of the tempest, and the distance of the clouds, but this tempest is not violent, and that the

cloud

Of the Air, Atmosphere, *&c.* 61

cloud is at a great distance, or high in the air, you may know by the length of time there is between your seeing the flash of lightning, and hearing the clap of thunder. Look, see how the sky opens to emit the fire; presently you will hear the thunder; for you know we see the fire from a gun at a distance long before we hear the report! There it is! and how tremendous!—These tempests always put me in mind of that beautiful passage in *Shakespear's King Lear*; where, when the good old King is out in a storm, and obliged to fly from his unnatural children, he says,

———— Let the great Gods,
That keep this dreadful thund'ring o'er our heads,
Find out their Enemies now. Tremble, thou wretch,
That hast within thee undivulged crimes
Unwhipt of justice! Hide thee, thou bloody hand,
Thou perjur'd, and thou simular of virtue,
That art incestuous! Caitiff, shake to pieces,
That under covert and convenient seeming
Has practised on man's life! Close pent-up guilt,
Rive your concealing continents, and ask
These dreadful summoners grace!————

This

This tempest will not give me leave to ponder
On things would hurt me more——

 Poor naked wretches, wheresoe'er you are,
That bide the pelting of this pitiless storm!
How shall your houseless heads, and unfed sides,
Your loop'd and widow'd raggedness defend
  you
From seasons such as these?—O, I have ta'en
Too little care of this! Tak physic, Pomp,
Expose thyself, to feel what wretches feel,
That thou mavst shake the superflux to them,
And shew the Heaven's more just.

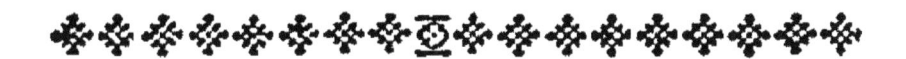

LECTURE IV.

Of MOUNTAINS, SPRINGS, RIVERS, and the SEA.

WE come now, says the Philosopher, to the consideration of things with which we are more intimately acquainted, but which are not, on that account, the less wonderful. How was that Mountain lifted up to the sky? How came this crystal Spring to bubble on its lofty brow, or that large River to flow from its massy side? But above all, how came this mighty body

body of water, the Sea, so collected together; and why and how was it impregnated with salt, seeing the fish and other animals taken out of it are perfectly fresh? These are questions not to be answered even by the Sages in Science. Here the Philosopher, at the end of his judgment, and lost in admiration, can only say with the Psalmist, *They that go down into the Sea, and occupy their business in the great waters, these men see the greatness of God, and his wonders in the deep.* Wonderful are thy works, O Lord, in judgment hast thou made them all!—The earth is full of thy greatness!

It is the business of Philosophy, however, to enquire into these things, though our enquiries are sometimes vain we shall therefore, in this Lecture give the best account we can of *Mountains, Springs, Rivers,* and the *Sea.*

The antients supposed that Mountains were originally occasioned by the Deluge, before which time they imagined that the earth was a perfect level, and a certain Abbot was taken into custody and punished for asserting that the earth was round; though there is so great a necessity for its being so, that according to the properties with which the Almighty has endowed the substances that compose the world, it could not conveniently subsist in any other form, for, not to mention the formation of rivers, which are generally occasioned by the mists that fall on the mountains, if the earth was not round it would be for ever covered with water: for it is, I think, supposed, that there is full as much water as earth, and as the water is specifically lighter than earth, that would be always uppermost, and we should have no dry land.

I protest, says Lady *Caroline*, I think you carry this argument too far, and seem to question the power of the Creator. How can you tell that the earth and water thus disposed would have that effect? From daily experience, Madam, says the Philosopher. Throw this stone into the moat and you will see it sink, or this clot of dirt, and it will fall to the bottom. But, says she, this is not always the case, for when I water my flowers the water sinks into the ground and disappears. That is because there is abundantly more earth than water, Madam, says he, and the earth being porous, or hollow, the water runs into the cavities and fills them;

but

but was you to keep on pouring out of the water-pot till all these crevices were full, you would find the water flow at top, and the garden mould, or earth, would remain at the bottom, for if you take a pint pot of earth, and another of water, and mix them ever so well together, the earth will in a little time subside or fall to the bottom, and the water will be seen at the top. This is to me a demonstration, Madam, and it is so far from calling in question the wisdom of God, that it is vindicating his wisdom in the works of Creation. So that you may perceive from hence, as well as from the motion of the heavenly bodies, that the earth is round, and that the ancients were in an error.

And with regard to Mountains, tho' the Deluge might throw up many, and much alter the face of the earth, yet from the great use mountains are of in collecting the waters of the atmosphere into springs and rivers, it is reasonable to suppose there were mountains even in the first age of the world.

If I am not mistaken, says Lady *Twilight*, it has been supposed, and by men of learning, that this irregularity of the earth's surface was occasioned by some
Comets,

Comets, striking against it, and this opinion, I know, put Lady *Lucy* and many others in great pain when the late Comet was expected. What say you to this, young Gentleman?

I am unable to answer for all the extravagant conceits and ridiculous follies of the human race, Madam, says he, and your Ladyship might as well expect me to give a reason for the poor soldier's prophesying an earthquake some time ago, and of the terrors of the people on that occasion, as to account for this. That the Earth has undergone amazing changes since its first formation, is, I think, evident from the contents of some mountains even in our own country, in which we find not only petrifactions in abundance, but the shells of sea fish, and even the bones of animals that were never inhabitants of this climate. At *Reading* in *Berkshire*, which is above forty miles from the sea, there is a stratum of oyster shells, which appear like real oysters, and are spread through a hill of considerable extent; they lie upon a chalky rock in a bed of sand, much resembling that of the sea, and the upper part of the hill, which is a loamy soil, is thirty or forty feet perpendicular above them; and at

Burton near *Petworth* in *Sussex*, was dug out of a pit, the bones or skeleton of an elephant. Numberless curiosities of this kind have been discovered here, (some of which I shall take particular notice of in my next course of Lectures) but I think there are few but what may be accounted for from the effects of the deluge, earthquakes, and subterraneous fires. Earthquakes at the bottom of the sea, for instance, have sometimes thrown up mountains or little islands, with the fish upon them, which have been covered by the sandy or loose earth giving way and falling over them. It is not long since an island was raised in this manner, in the *Archipelago*, of ten miles circumference, the hills of which abound with oysters not yet petrified, and which are much larger than those taken on the coast; whence we may conclude, that they were thrown up from the deepest part of the sea. Sea-fish have been also found in other mountains, some of which have been petrified, while others have been found with the flesh only browned or mummied.

And from the amazing quantity of fire contained in the earth, and of the subterranean air rarified thereby, great alterations

tions muſt have been made in its ſurface, in the courſe of ſo many years.

Very well, ſays Lady *Caroline*, and ſo you are going to turn the earth into a hot-bed, and I ſuppoſe, we who are its inhabitants, are by and by to be complimented with the title of muſhrooms and cucumbers, or perhaps pumpkins. This is fine philoſophy, indeed. Have patience, my dear, ſays the Marchioneſs. Patience, Ma'am, returned Lady *Caroline*, why I hope your Ladyſhip would not have me believe that we have a furnace of fire under us? I don't know, Madam, whether it be immediately under us or not, replied the little Philoſopher; but that there are a number of theſe furnaces in the earth is beyond diſpute, and is evidently proved by the great number of burning mountains, which are continually ſending up flames, attended with large ſtones and metallic ſubſtances. I am ſorry his Grace of *Galaxy* is gone, Madam, for he would have ſet you right in this particular, which, pardon me, I ſhall not attempt, ſince I find my veracity ſo much queſtioned. The company all laughed at the Philoſopher in a *pit*, but the Marchioneſs took up the matter, and ſoon put an end to the diſpute

Of Mountains, Springs, &c. 69

pute. She blamed Lady *Caroline* for offering to decide upon a point which she did not understand, and then turning to the young gentleman, told him, that patience ought to be a principal ingredient in the character of a Philosopher upon which Lady *Caroline* and he compoſed their difference with a mutual ſmile, and after aſking the Marchioneſs pardon for betraying too much warmth, even in the cauſe of truth, he told Lady *Caroline*, ſhe ſhould have ſome account of theſe mountains from the beſt authority, when, taking a book out of his pocket, he read as follows:

"The moſt famous of theſe mountains is *Ætna* in *Sicily*, whoſe eruptions of flame and ſmoke are diſcovered at a great diſtance, by thoſe that ſail on the *Mediterranean*, even as far as the harbour of *Malta*, which is forty *German* miles from the ſhore of *Sicily*. Though fire and ſmoke are continually vomited up by it, yet at ſome particular time it rages with greater violence. In the year 1536 it ſhook all *Sicily*, from the firſt to the twelfth of *May*; after that, there was heard a moſt horrible bellowing and cracking, as if great guns had been fired; there were a great many houſes over-

G   thrown

thrown throughout the whole island. When this storm had continued about eleven days, the ground opened in several places, and dreadful gapings appeared here and there, from which issued forth fire and flame with great violence, which in four days consumed and burnt up every thing that was within five leagues of Ætna. A little after the funnel, which is on the top of the mountain, disgorged a great quantity of hot embers and ashes, for three whole days together, which were not only dispersed throughout the whole island, but also carried beyond sea to *Italy*; and several ships that were sailing to *Venice*, at two hundred leagues distance, suffered damage. *Facellus* hath given us an historical account of the eruptions of this mountain, and says, that the bottom of it is one hundred leagues in circuit.

"HECLA, a mountain in *Iceland*, rages sometimes with as great violence as Ætna, and casts out great stones. The imprisoned fire often, by want of vent, causes horrible sounds, like lamentations and howlings, which make some credulous people think it the place of Hell, where the souls of the wicked are tormented.

"VESUVIUS

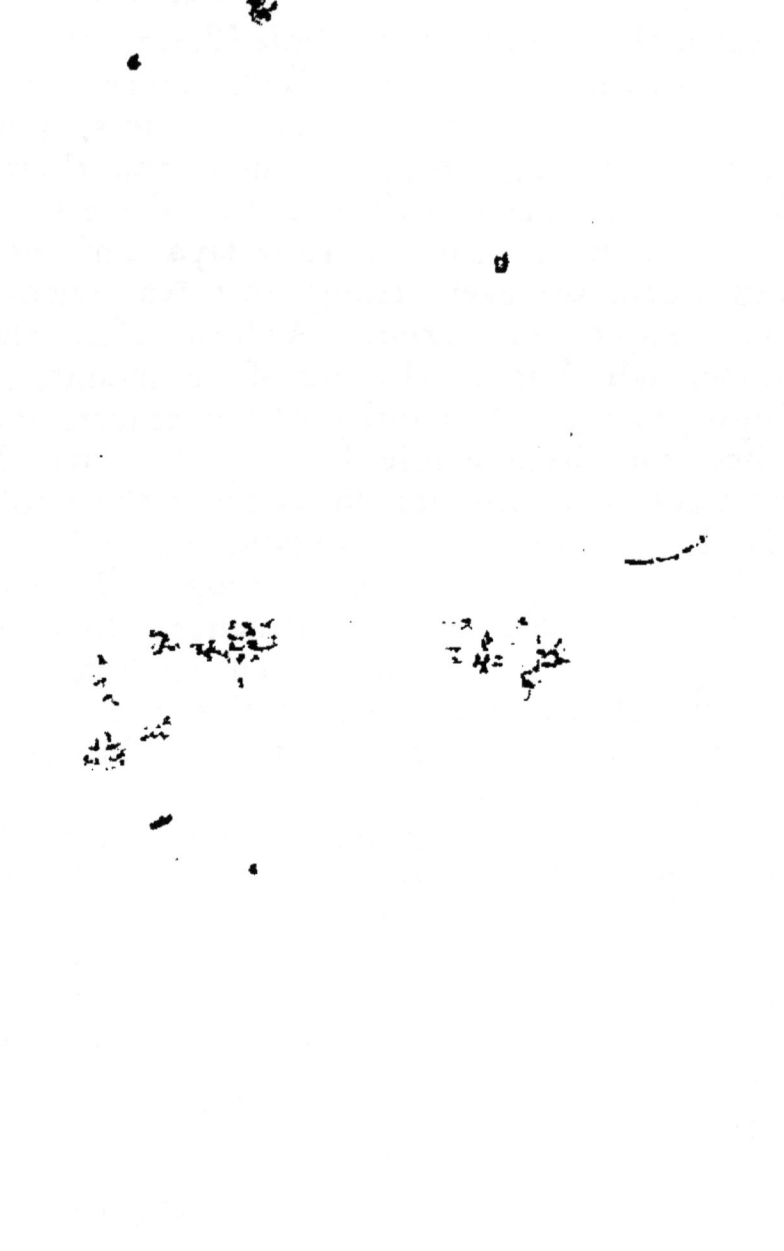

Mount Vesuvius

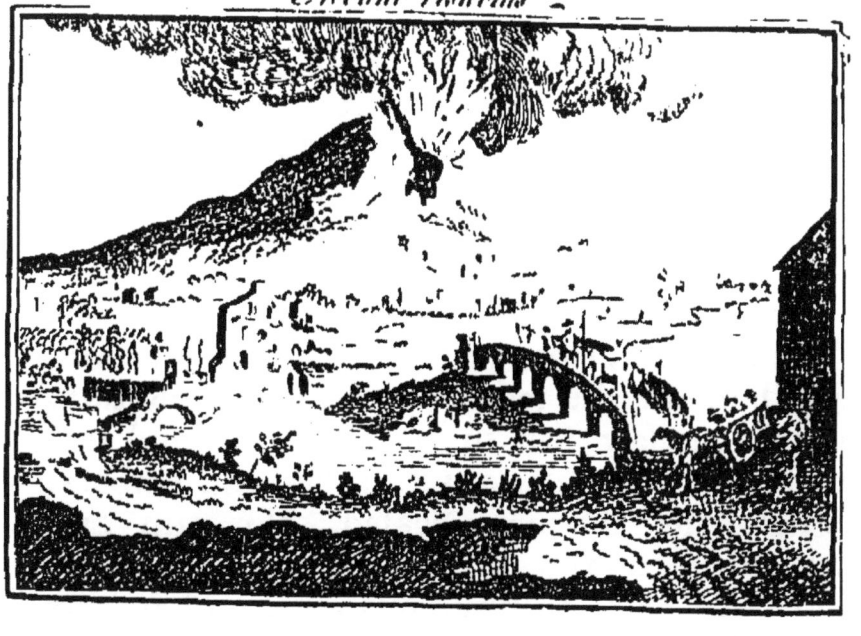

Of Mountains, Springs, &c.

"Vesuvius in *Campania*, not far from the town of *Naples*, though it be planted with most fruitful vines, and at other times yieldeth the best *Muscadel* wines, yet it is very often annoyed with violent eruptions. *Dion Cassius* relates, that in the reign of *Vespasian*, there was such a dreadful eruption of impetuous flames, that great quantities of ashes and sulphureous smoke were not only carried to *Rome* by the wind, but also beyond the *Mediterranean*, into *Africa*, and even into *Egypt*. Moreover, birds were suffocated in the air, and fell down dead upon the ground, and fishes perished in the neighbouring waters, which were made hot and infected by it. There happened another eruption in *Martial*'s time, which he elegantly describes in one of his *Epigrams*, and laments the sad change of the mountain, which he saw first in its verdure, and immediately after black with ashes and embers. When the burning ceased, the rain and dew watered the surface of the mountain, and made these sulphureous ashes and embers fruitful, so that they produced a large increase of excellent wine, but when the mountain begun to burn again, and to disgorge fire and smoke afresh, (which sometimes hap-

happened within a few years) then were the neighbouring fields burnt up, and the highways made dangerous to travellers.

"A mountain in *Java*, not far from the town of *Panacuja*, in the year 1586, was shattered to pieces by a violent eruption of glowing sulphur, (though it had never burnt before) whereby (as it was reported) ten thousand people perished in the under-land fields. It threw up large stones and cast them as far as *Pancras*, and continued for three days to throw out so much black smoke, mixed with flames and hot embers, that it darkened the face of the Sun, and made the day appear as dark as the night."

There are a great number of other mountains, or, (as your Ladyship is pleased to call them) furnaces in the known world, which I shall take some notice of in my next course of Lectures.

We come now to the consideration of Springs, which are occasioned principally, we may suppose, by the water exhaled from the sea, rivers, lakes, and marshy places; and, forming clouds, are dispersed by the winds. These clouds, when they are so collected together as to become too heavy to be supported by the air, fall down in rain

rain to water the herbs and plants, but those that are lighter, being driven aloft in the air, dash against the mountains, and to them give up their contents in small particles; whence entering the crevices, they descend till they meet together, and form Springs, and this is the reason why we have such plenty of Springs in mountainous countries, and few or none in those that are flat. And you may observe, that it frequently rains in hilly countries, when it is clear and fine in the valleys beneath, for the air in the valleys is dense enough to support the clouds and keep them suspended; but being driven up among mountains, where, in consequence of their height, the air is so much lighter, they descend in mists or such small drops of rain that will not run off, as is the case in a heavy rain, but sink into the crevices of the earth in the manner already mentioned. Now that a great part of this water is exhaled from the sea, may be known by the extraordinary rains and great dews which fall upon islands that are surrounded by the sea. But some Springs, it is reasonable to suppose, have their source from the ocean, since those which we meet with near the sea, are generally somewhat salt or brackish.

These

These springs, thus formed by the mists on mountains and the rain meeting together, form little rivulets or brooks, and those again uniting compose large rivers, which empty themselves into the sea; and in this manner the water, exhaled from the sea by the sun, is returned to it again, for Providence has established such wise laws or regulations for the world, that no part of the elements can be annihilated. But the very large rivers must have some other source besides the springs formed by the mists, dews, and rains, since these seem insufficient to support their prodigious discharge; it is therefore no improbable conjecture to suppose, that they have some communication with the sea, and that the salt water is purified and rendered sweet by passing through the sand, gravel, and crevices of the earth. And this I shall endeavour to prove in my next course of lectures.

Lakes are collections of water contained in the cavities of the surface of the earth, some of which are said to be stagnant, and made up of the waste water that flows, after rain or snow, from the adjacent countries, and these must be unwholesome. Other Lakes are supplied by rivers, the contents of which they receive and convey under ground,

ground, to form other springs and rivers; others, again, are fed by springs which arise in the Lake itself, and some (as that of *Haerlem*, and other salt Lakes) have a communication, it is supposed, with the sea, whence they receive their waters, and afterwards discharge them by subterranean streams.

The sea is a great collection of water in the deep valleys of the earth, I say, in the deep valleys; for if there were not prodigious cavities in the earth to contain this amazing quantity of water, thus collected together, the whole surface of the globe would be overflowed, for the water being lighter than the earth, would be above the earth, as the air is above the water.

Now you speak of the Sea, says the Marchioness, I wish you would tell me why the Sea-water is always salt. Madam, replied he, I wish I could, but it is beyond the reach of my Philosophy, and, indeed, I believe, of any Philosophy whatever. You might as well ask me, why there is water, as why there is salt in the water, which indeed seems almost as much an element as that: And I have often thought, from the prodigious quantity of salt distributed in the earth

earth and water, that it must have qualities that we know not of, and answer purposes in the scale of Being with which we are unacquainted.

The most remarkable quality in the Sea, next to its saltness, is that motion or rising and falling of the water, which we call *tides*, and which is occasioned by the attraction of the Moon, for that part of the water in the great ocean, which is nearest the Moon, being strongly attracted, is raised higher than the rest, and the part opposite to it, on the contrary side, being least attracted, is also higher than the rest. And these two opposite sides of the surface of the water, in the great ocean, following the motion of the Moon from East to West, and striking against the large coasts of the Continent, from thence rebound back again, and so make *floods* and *ebbs*, in narrow seas and rivers, at a distance from the great ocean. This also accounts for the periodical times of the *tides*, and for their constantly following the course of the Moon.

LECTURE

LECTURE V.

Of MINERALS, VEGETABLES, and ANIMALS.

COULD a Philosopher condescend to envy the Great, it would not be for their sumptuous palaces and numerous attendants, but for the means and opportunities they have of enquiring into the secrets of Nature, and contemplating the wonderful works of God. There is no subject so worthy of a rational creature, except that of promoting the happiness of Mankind; and none, except that, can give a man of refined taste, and good understanding, so much real satisfaction. But it is our misfortune, that few engage in those enquiries, but men of small estate, whose circumstances will not permit them to spare the time, nor support the expence of travelling, which is often necessary to obtain the knowledge they seek after, and for the want of which they are obliged to depend on the relations of those, who have not, perhaps, been so accurate or so faithful as they ought. Considering the quantity of foreign drugs that are used in *Britain*, it is amazing how little even those who deal in them know of the matter, so little, indeed, that they cannot tell where they grow, or how they are found or manufactured, are unable to distinguish the genuine from the fictitious, and may therefore, through mistake, often substitute the one for the other. Health and Life are of too much consequence to be trifled with, yet these are neglected, while Fashion, Dress, and Diversions, are sought after throughout the world. This is a melancholy consideration; but this, you'll say, is no part of our Lecture, therefore we shall drop a subject which has thrust itself, as it were, into our way, and speak of the contents of the earth, and its products and inhabitants. For this globe, besides the earth and water which are necessary for the production and support of Plants and Animals, contain other materials which have been found useful to Man. That Reflecting Telescope, this Gold Watch, and Lady *Caroline*'s Diamond Ear rings, were all dug out of the Earth, at least the materials were there found of which these things are composed.

Those sorts of earth which with the assistance of rain produce Vegetables or
Plants

Plants in such abundance, are *common mould, loam, clay,* and *sandy soils.* There are earths, also, that are different from these, and which are used in medicine, as the *Japan earth, Armenian Bole, &c.*

The barren parts of the earth, are, for the most part, *sand, gravel, chalk,* and *rocks*; for these produce nothing, unless they have earth mixed with them.—Of barren sands there are various kinds, though their chief difference is in their colour, for the sand which we throw on paper, to prevent blotting, and that the maid throws on the floor, are both composed of little irregular stones, without any earth, and of such there are large desarts in some parts of the world, and one in particular, where *Cambyses,* an Eastern Monarch, lost an army of 50,000 men. Sure, says Lady *Caroline,* you must mistake, Sir. How was it possible for a whole army to be lost in that manner? Why, Madam, returned the Philosopher, the wind, as it frequently does in those parts, raised the sands and clouds, for many days together, and the whole army was smothered. And if you read the life of *Alexander the Great,* you'll find, Madam, that his army was in great danger, when he crossed the same desart, in his frantick expedition to visit the temple of

his

his pretended Father *Jupiter Ammon.*—But we return to our subject.

Besides these materials which compose the surface of the earth, if we dig deeper, we frequently find bodies very different from those we discover near the surface, and these, because they are discovered by digging into the bowels of the earth, are called by the common name of *Fossils*; though under this head are included all *metals*, and *metallic ores*, *minerals*, or *half metals*, stones of various sorts, *petrifactions*, or *animal* substances turned into stone; and many other bodies which have a texture between stone and earth, as, *oker* of several sorts, with one of which the farmers colour their sheep; *black lead*, with which are made those pencils that we use for drawing; and some kinds of *chalk*, *sea-coal*, and other bodies that are harder than earth, and yet not of the consistency of perfect stone.

Of *stones* there is an amazing variety. They are classed by Naturalists under two heads, that is to say, *spars*, and *crystals*; and by others into *vulgar* and *precious stones*. Some of the most considerable, both for beauty and use, are *marble, alabaster, porphyry, granite, free-stone, &c.* Flints, agates, cornelians, and *pebbles*, under which kind

kind are placed the *precious stones*, otherwise called *gems* or *jewels*, which are only *stones* of an excessive hardness, and which, when cut and polished, have an extraordinary lustre. The most valuable of these are *diamonds, rubies, sapphires, amethysts, emeralds, topazes,* and *opals*.

But there are other stones, which though void of beauty, may, perhaps, have more virtue than many of those already mentioned; such as the *loadstone*, which has the property of directing the needle in the mariners compass always to or near the North Pole; by which means we are enabled to sail even in the darkest night. Such also are *whetstones*, with which we sharpen our knives and other edge tools, *limestones, talk, calamine,* or *lapis calaminaris*, and many others.

Besides the bodies already mentioned, there are also found in the earth a variety of salts, such as *rock salt*, or *sal gem, vitriol, nitre,* and many others.

The *minerals, marcasites,* or *semi-metals,* as they are called by the Chemists, are *antimony, zinc, bismuth,* &c. These are not inflammable, ductile, or malleable, but are hard and brittle, and may be reduced to powder; and the first, after melting, may be calcined by fire.

H   *Mercury*

Mercury, or *quickfilver*, has generally been claffed with *femi metals*, and indeed, fometimes among the metals, but I think it ought not to be claffed under either of thefe heads, but confidered feparately; as alfo fhould *brimftone*, though it be a part of the compofition of *crude antimony*.

Ores are thofe kinds of earth which are dug out of mines, and that contain in them metallic particles from whence metals are extracted.

Metals are diftinguifhed from other bodies by their weight, fufibility or melting in the fire, and their malleability, or giving way, and extending under the ftroke of the hammer without breaking in pieces. Thefe are fix, *viz gold, filver, copper, tin, lead,* and *iron*, which laft is the moft valuable of them all. They are feldom or never found in any part of the earth but what is mountainous, which, by the way, in fome meafure proves what we ventured to affert in a former Lecture, *viz* that there were mountains before the Deluge; for that there were metals before the Deluge appears by what is faid in Holy Writ concerning *Tubal Cain*, who wrought in brafs, *&c.* and was the inventor of organs.

All *ftones, minerals,* and *metals,* are fuppofed

posed to grow organically in the earth from their proper seeds, as vegetables do on the earth's surface. And what sort of bodies are to be found deeper in the earth, I mean towards its centre, is unknown to us, for we can only make ourselves acquainted with the fossi's contained in its shell, and the vegetables and animals on its surface, whose nature and properties alone are, indeed, too many to be discovered by human sagacity.

Of Vegetables or Plants.

The Vegetables or Plants growing on the earth may be divided into three classes, I me in those of *herbs, shrubs*, and *trees*.

Herbs, are those sorts of vegetables whose stalks are soft, and have no wood in them, as *parsley, lettuce, violets, pinks, grass, nettles, thistles*, and an infinate number of others.

Shrubs are those plants which, though woody, never grow into trees, but bow down their branches near the earth's surface, such are those plants that produce *roses, honeysuckles, gooseberries, currants*, and the like.

But *Trees* shoot up in one great stem or body, and rise to a considerable distance from the ground before they spread their branches, as may be seen by the *oak*, the *beech*, the elm,

elm, the *ash*, the *fir*, the *walnut-tree*, *cherry-tree*, and others. From the bodies of trees we have our timber for building, and of the oak tree in particular for ship building, no timber being so tough, strong, and durable as old *English* oak, nor does any tree, perhaps, yield more timber; for there was one lately sold for forty pounds, from *Langley* woods, belonging to the Bishop of *Salisbury*, which measured six feet two inches in diameter, contained ten tons of timber, and was supposed to be a thousand years old.

"From a small acorn see the oak arise
Supremely tall, and tow'ring to the skies!
Queen of the groves, her stately head she rears,
Her bulk encreasing by the length of years;
Now ploughs the sea, a warlike gallant ship,
Whilst in her womb destructive thunder sleep:
Hence BRITAIN boasts her wide extensive reign,
And by th' expanded acorn rules the Main."

The most considerable parts of plants are the *root*, the *stalk*, the *leaves*, the *flowers*, and the *seed*, most of them have these several parts, though there are some, indeed, that have no stalk, as the *aloe*; others that have no leaves, as *savine*, and others that have no flowers, as *fern*. But I think there are none without *root* or *seed*, though some say that *fern* is an exception as to the last.

What most excites our wonder with respect

to plants (and what, indeed, has been the subject of much dispute among the learned) is their *nourishment* and *propagation*.—This, says Master *Blossom*, I have often heard my father discourse upon when I have been in the garden with him, but as what he said has escaped my memory, I should be glad, Sir, if you would tell me how they receive their nourishment, and how their species are propagated. A disquisition of this nature, says the little Philosopher, would take up too much of your time, and could not be understood without reciting many experiments and observations that have been made by the learned, I shall, therefore, defer the consideration of it till my next course of Lectures. I see no reason for that, says Master *Wilson*, nor to me does there appear any difficulty in the affair. Why, they receive their nourishment from the earth, don't they? And you sow the seeds of the old plants and they produce new ones.

You are too apt, Master *Wilson*, says the Philosopher, to talk about things you don't understand. The earth has not, perhaps, so much to do with the nourishment of plants as is generally imagined; for, without water, and particularly rain water and dew, there would be but little increase in vegeta-

bles

bles of any kind; and this you may know by the languid state of plants in a dry season, though watered ever so often from the river or well. This is known also by the small quantity of earth which is taken up in the growth of plants, for both Mr. *Boyle* and Dr. *Woodward* raised several plants in earth watered with rain or spring water, and even distilled water, and upon weighing the dry earth, both before and after the production of the plants, they have found that very little of it was diminished or taken up by the plant. Taken up by the plant, says Lady *Caroline*, in some surprise, why you don't imagine there is earth in herbs and trees? Indeed I do, Madam, replied the little Philosopher, and have already hinted as much in what was said on the four elements, and at the same time told your Ladyship, if I mistake not, how it might be extracted from the plant, which was, by burning the plant to ashes, and washing off the salts, as your laundry maid does when she makes lye, for when these salts are washed away the remainder will be earth

If the earth contributes so little towards the production of plants, says Master *Blyth*, the water, I apprehend, must be a good deal concerned, and that is evident from the quantity

Of VEGETABLES. 87

quantity of water which most plants require to keep them in a state of health and vigour. Your observations, says the Philosopher, deserves some notice, but how will you account for the growth of plants in sandy desarts where it seldom rains, and of plants too, that contain juices in great abundance; for God Almighty, for the preservation of his creatures, has caused those wonderful plants to grow in such barren desarts to supply, in some measure, the want of water; and some are so constructed as to hold great quantities of water for the use of animals. This is the case of the ground Pine*, which, though it seems to grow like a fungus or excrescence on the branch of a tree, often contains a pint or a quart of sweet water for the birds, beasts, and even men, to refresh themselves within the sultry climates where they abound. But a plant may hold much water for the subsistence of animals, and yet not subsist in water itself, and that this is the case experience testifies. Dr. *Wood-ward* puts a plant of *spearmint*, which weighed 27 grains, into a phial

---

* For a more particular account of this plant, we must refer our readers to the *Christian Magazine*, Numb. II. where it is introduced with suitable reflections to demonstrate the wonders of God in the works of creation.

of

of water, where it stood 77 days, and in that time drank up 2558 grains of spring water. And then being taken out weighed 42 grains, so that the increase was only 15 grains, which is not a hundredth part of the water expended.—We are therefore to look for other principles of vegetables than what are generally known, but this I shall consider in my next course of Lectures.

What the plant can obtain by the earth, water, and otherwise for its nourishment, is generally supposed to be received by the fibres of the roots, and conveyed by the stalk or body of the plant up into the branches and leaves through small tubes, and then returned by the bark to the root again; so that there is a constant circulation of vital fluids in plants as well as in animals. But I am inclined to think, that a great part of the nourishment of plants is received by the pores of the leaves and skin or bark, as well as from the root, else how happens it that plants are so much refreshed by the dew?

Plants also require air for their nourishment, as well as a circulation of these alimentary juices; for they respire as well as animals, and for that respiration require fresh air, and even exercise, since we know that plants, that are always confined in a close room,

Of Vegetables. 89

room, will never rise to perfection. And that they perspire as well as animals is evident, from the instance of the *mint* growing in spring-water above-mentioned; for if not a hundredth part of the water taken up by that plant became a part of the plant itself, all the rest must be perspired through the pores, or little imperceptible holes in the skin and leaves. This calls to my mind, says Lady *Caroline*, a charge my Lord Marquis gave me, which was, never to sit in the *yew arbor*; for the matter perspired by the yew-tree, says he, is noxious, and will make you ill, and I believe that was the reason of his Lordship's ordering that old arbor to be demolished.

But pray, Sir, why and in what manner can plants perspire? For the same reason, Madam, and in the same manner, perhaps, that animals do, returned the Philosopher. It is occasioned, probably, by heat; for we know that they perspire abundantly more in summer than in winter; nay, when this vegetative principle has been long checked by cold, it breaks out with such force, when warm weather comes on, that it is no uncommon thing, in the cold northern countries, to see the trees covered with snow one week, and with blossoms the next.

Plants

Plants are propagated different ways, but the most general method is by seed. Some plants, however, are raised by a part of the root of the old plant set in the ground, as potatoes; others, by new roots propagated from the old ones, as *hyacinths*, and *tulips*; others, by cutting off branches and putting them into the ground, which will there take root and grow, as *vines*; and others are propagated by grafting and budding, or inoculation. But what I represented as most mysterious, and indeed for the subject of a Lecture in my next Course, is the Sexes of plants; for many sorts have both male and female organs and the one will not flourish and increase without the aid of the other.

Of Animals.

We are now to speak of the Animals that inhabit the earth, which are naturally divided into *Men* and *Brutes*.

Of Men, there seem to be four different sorts.—Nay, don't be frightened, Lady *Caroline!*—Sir, says she, I should have made no objection, had you said four hundred, provided you had distinguished them according to their different dispositions —— True, Madam, says the Philosopher, or according to their different features, and then you

you might have said four hundred thousand; for it is very true, Madam, tho' very wonderful, that out of four hundred thousand faces you will not find two exactly alike; and but for this miraculous and gracious providence in God, the world would have been all in confusion. But the division I would willingly make of men, Lady *Caroline*, is that of *white, tawny, black*, and *red*; and these you will allow are, with respect to colour, essentially different. Most of the *Europeans*, and some of the *Asiatic* are *white*; the *Africans* on the coast of the *Mediterranean* sea are *tawny*; those on the coast of *Guinea black*; and the original *Americans red*, or of a red copper colour: How they came so is only known to their Maker; and therefore I beg you would spare yourselves the trouble of asking me any question on that head.

Brutes may be divided into four classes; that is to say, 1. *Aerial*, or such as have wings and fly in the air, as *birds, wasps, flies*, &c. 2. *Terrestrial*, or those which are confined to the earth, as *quadrupeds*, or four-footed beasts; *reptiles*, which have many feet; and *serpents*, which have no feet at all. 3. *Aquatick*, or those that live in the water, as *fish* of all kinds, whether they are covered with scales or shells, or are, like the *eel*, without either. 4. *Amphibious*, or those that can live for a long time either upon the earth, or in the water, as *otters, alligators, turtles*, &c. I say for a long time, because I apprehend, that the use of both these elements are necessary for the subsistence of those animals; and that though they can live for a considerable time upon land in the open air, or as long in the water, excluded in a manner from air, yet they would languish and die, if confined entirely either to the one or the other of these elements.

In this division of animals we are to observe, however, that there are some which cannot be considered under either class, being, as it were, of a middle nature and partaking of two kinds; thus *bats* seem to be partly beasts and partly birds. Some *reptiles*, likewise, and some of the water animals, want one or more of the five senses with which other animals are endowed, as *worms, cockles, oysters*, &c. If I mistake not, says Lady *Caroline*, I have seen the animals divided into different classes in books of Natural History, and described under the heads of *beasts, birds, fishes*, and *insects*. Very true, Madam, says the Philosopher; but the present method suits my present purpose the best, and can make no alteration in the

nature

nature of things; however, as I have not yet mentioned the word *infects*, tho' they are included in my division of animals, it may be necessary for me to observe, that they are so called from a separation in their bodies, by which they are seemingly divided into two parts, those parts being only joined together by a small ligament, as in *flies*, *wasps*, &c. And as some of these *insects* undergo different changes, and in time become quite different animals, I shall consider them more particularly in my next Course of Lectures, not having time for it at present; for it is a field that is full of wonders, and ought to be examined with great attention. There is something so amazing and miraculous in the transformation of infects, that I am lost in reflection whenever the subject strikes my mind, and sometimes inclined to think that other animals may undergo some such change. Who, that had not made the observation, would think, Madam, that this *grub* crawling or rather sleeping here, would by and by become a fine *butterfly*, decked out in all the gaudy colours of the rainbow; or that this *silkworm* should be capable of assuming so many different forms? And is it not altogether as miraculous, that if some animals are cut in pieces, every separate piece or part of the original animal will become one entire animal of itself? Yet that the *polype* or *polypus* is endowed with this property has been demonstrated; and I have here one that was divided into several parts some time ago, which parts are now become distinct and perfect *polypes* and alive, as you may see by viewing them through this microscope.

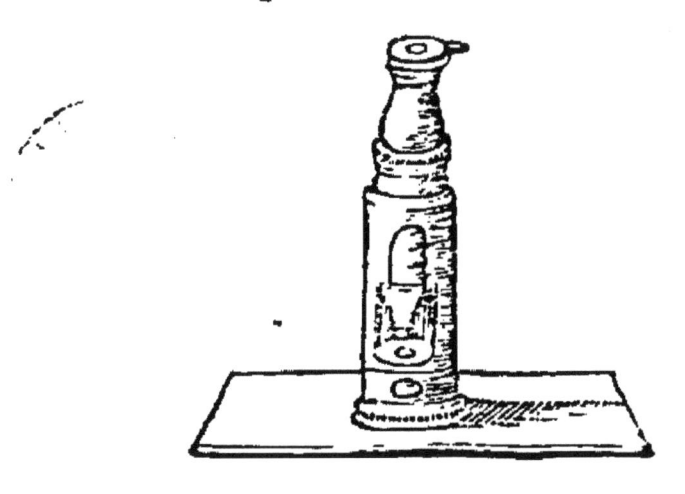

But the sagacity and acute senses of some of the animals (in which they seem to exceed man) are altogether as surprizing, as I shall demonstrate in my next Course. In your next course, says Master *Wilson*, why don't you do it now? Peace, prithee, *Tom*, says the Philosopher, learn this first, and then I'll talk to you about *beavers* building of houses,

houses; *bees* forming themselves into a society, and chusing a Queen to govern them; *birds* knowing the latitude and longitude, and sailing over sea through vast tracts of air, from one country to another, without the use of any compass, and of other things, which are sufficient, I think, to lower the pride of man, and make even Philosophers blush at their own ignorance.—And now, Lady *Caroline*, prepare to here a few hard words, and I will finish this Lecture. But why must it be finished in an unintelligible manner? says the Lady. Because I cannot deliver what I am going to say, Madam, without making use of the terms of art, says he, and those I must desire your Ladyship, and the rest of the good company, to learn from Mr. *Newbery*'s Pocket Dictionary, or some other book of that kind.

All animals receive their food at the mouth, and most animals, but especially those of the human kind, chew it there till it is intimately mixed with the saliva or spittle, and thereby prepared for the easier and better digestion in the stomach. When the stomach has digested the food, it is thence conveyed into the *guts* (pardon the expression, Ladies, for I cannot avoid it) through which it is moved gently by what is called the *peristaltick motion*; as it passes there, the *chyle*, which is the nutritive part, is separated by the *lacteal veins*, from the excrementitious parts, and by them conveyed into the blood, with which it circulates, and is concocted into blood also; and this circulation is thus performed. The blood being, by the *vena cava*, brought into the right ventricle of the heart, by the contraction of that muscle, is forced into the *pulmonary artery* of the lungs, where the air, which is continually inspired or drawn in by the lungs, mixes with and enlivens it; and from thence the blood, being conveyed by the *pulmonary vein* into the left ventricle of the heart, the contraction of the heart forces it out, and by the arteries distributes it into all parts of the body, from whence it returns by the veins to the right ventricle of the heart, to pursue the same course again, in order to communicate life and heat to every part of this wonderful machine, the body. But this is not all; for, according to Anatomists, some part of the blood, in the course of its circulation, goes to the head, where a portion of it is separated by the brain, and concocted into *animal spirits*, which are distributed by the nerves, and impart sense and motion throughout the body. The instruments

struments of motion, however, are the muscles; the fibres or small threads whereof, contracting themselves, move the different parts of the body; which in some of them is done by the direction of the mind, and called *voluntary motion*; but, in others, the mind seems not to be concerned, and therefore these motions are called *involuntary*.

This is the progress of animal life; by which you will perceive that a man may, even at home, and within himself, see the Wonders of God in the Works of Creation.

We have now finished our survey of the Universe, and considered these great masses of matter, the Stars and Planets; but particularly our earth and its inhabitants, all which large bodies are made up of inconceivable small *bodies*, or *atoms*. And by the figure, texture, bulk, and motion of these insensible *corpuscles*, or infinitely small bodies, all the phenomena of large bodies may be explained.

LECTURE VI.

Of the FIVE SENSES *of* MAN, *and of his* UNDERSTANDING.

AT our next meeting there was a great deal of good company, who came to hear the *Boys Philosophy*, as they called it; on which account I could observe that Master *Telescope* took less pains to be understood by the young Gentlemen and Ladies, and addressed himself more particularly to those of greater abilities.

As the company came in laughing, and affected to talk, and behaved in a supercilious manner, (which even some great personages do in these our days of refinement) he stood silent, till my Lord Marquis desired him to open the Lecture; upon which he bowed to his Lordship and the rest of the company, and began, but had scarcely spoken three words before he was interrupted by Sir *Harry*, he therefore stopped for some time, and then began again, but the tongue of the young Baronet soon silenced him, and he stood without speaking a considerable time. On this the company looked at each other,

and

and the Marquis bad him go on. My dear, says the Marchioness, how can you expect this young Gentleman to read a long Lecture, when you know that Sir *Harry*, who loves to hear himself talk of all things, has not patience to support so much taciturnity? Why, Madam, says the Ambassador of *Bantam* (who came in with the Marquis) I thought we had all been assembled to hear this Lecture. That was indeed the intention of our meeting says the Marchioness; but I hope your Excellency knows the polite world better, than to expect people should be so old fashioned as to behave on these occasions, with any sort of good manners or decorum. In my country, says the Ambassador, all the company keep a profound silence at these meetings. It may be so, replied the Marchioness; but I assure your Excellency, it is not the custom here. Why, Sir, I have been often interrupted in the middle of a fine air, at an Oratorio, by a Gentleman whistling a hornpipe, and, at the Rehearsal at St. *Paul*'s, it is no uncommon thing to hear both Gentlemen and Ladies laugh louder than the organ. Hush, Madam, says the Marquis, if your friends and neighbours are fools, you ought not to expose them, and especially to foreigners.

Take

Take care, while you condemn this unpolite behaviour in others, that you don't run into it yourself. *Politeness* is the art of being always agreeable in company, it can therefore seldom deal in *sarcasm* or *irony*; because it should never do any thing to abridge the happiness of others; and you see, my Dear, you have made Sir *Harry* uneasy, for he blushes. The company laughed at Sir *Harry*, who joined them, and being determined to hold his tongue, our Philosopher thus proceeded.

After the cursory view of nature, which was concluded in my last Lecture, it may not be amiss to examine our own faculties, and see by what means we acquire and treasure up a knowledge of these things; and this is done, I apprehend, by means of the *senses*, the operations of the *mind*, and the *memory*; which last may be called the storehouse of the *understanding*. The first time little Master is brought to a looking-glass, he thinks he has found a new play-mate, and calls out *Little boy! Little boy!* for having never seen his own face before, it is no wonder that he should not know it. Here is the idea, therefore, of something new acquired by *sight*.—Presently the father, and mother, and nurse come forward to partake of the child's

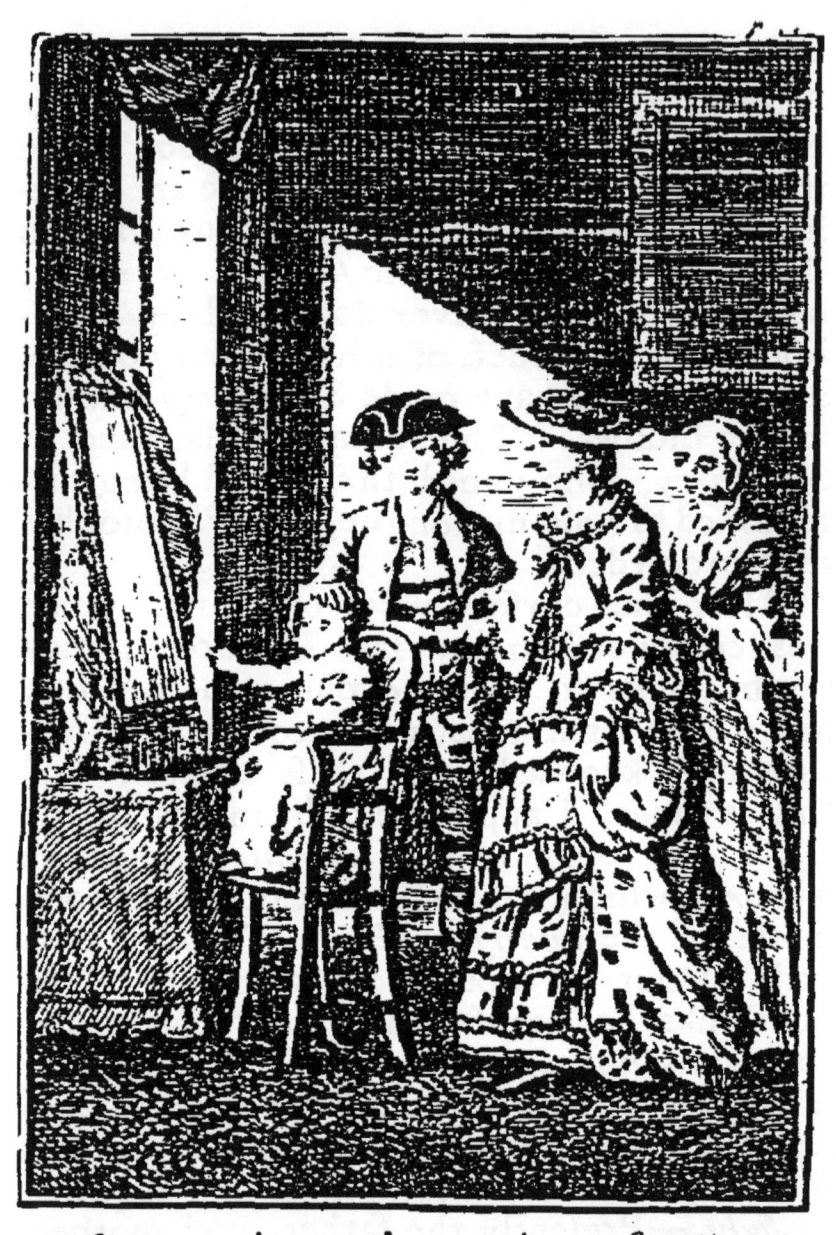

Aboy finds himself in the Glass.

child's diversion. Upon seeing these figures in the glass with whom he is so well acquainted, he immediately calls out, *There, Papa! there, Mamma! there, Nurse!* And now the *mind* begins to operate; for feeling his father's hand on his own head, and seeing it on the little boy's head in the glass, he cries, *There me!* Now this transaction is lodged in the *memory*, which, whenever a looking-glass is mentioned, will give back to the mind this idea of its reflecting objects.

The whole company were pleased with this familiar demonstration; but Sir *Harry* asked how he came of all things to make use of a looking-glass? Because, Sir, says he, it is an object with which some people are the most intimately acquainted ——As Sir *Harry* is an egregious fop, this reply produced a loud laugh, and master *Telescope* was looked upon to be a *Wit* as well as a *Philosopher*. however, I am inclined to think the expression was accidental, and not intended to hit Sir *Harry*, because I know his good sense would not permit him to treat an elder and superior in that manner — The laugh being a little subsided, our Philosopher thus proceeded on his Lecture.

All our ideas, therefore, are obtained either by *sensation* or *reflection*, that is to say,

say, by means of our five senses, as *seeing, hearing, smelling, tasting,* and *touching,* or by the *operations* of the *mind.*

Before you proceed farther, says the Countess of *Twilight,* you should, I think, explain to the company what is meant by the term *idea.* That, I apprehend, is sufficiently explained by what was said about the looking glass, says the Philosopher; but if your Ladyship requires another definition you shall have it. By an *idea,* then, I mean that *image* or *picture,* Madam, which is formed in the *mind* of any thing which we have *seen,* or even *heard talk of,* for the mind is so adroit and ready at this kind of *painting,* that a town, for instance, is no sooner mentioned, but the *imagination* shapes it into form and presents it to the *memory.* None of the company, I presume, have ever seen *Dresden,* yet there is not one, perhaps, but has formed, or conceived in his mind, some *idea* or *picture* of that unhappy place. Not one of us ever saw the *Nabob*'s prodigious army and elephants, yet we have all formed to ourselves a *picture* of their running away from a small party of our brave countrymen, led against them by the gallant and courageous Colonel *Clive.* When we read in the news-papers a description of a *sea engagement,*

gagement, or of the taking of *Louisbourg, Quebec*, or any other important fortress, the mind immediately gives us a *picture* of the *transaction*, and we see our valiant officers issuing their orders, and their intrepid men furling their sails, firing their guns, scaling the walls, and driving their foes before them. To pursue this subject a little farther—No man has ever seen a *dragon*, a *griffin*, or a *fairy*; yet every one has formed in his mind a *picture image*, or, in other words, an *idea*, of these imaginary beings—Now when this *idea* or *image* is formed in the mind from a view of the object itself, it may be called an *adequate* or *real idea*, but when it is conceived in the mind without seeing the object, it is an *inadequate* or *imaginary idea*

I shall begin my discourse of the Senses with that of the SIGHT, says he, because, as Mr. *Addison* observes, the *sight* is the most perfect and pleasing of them all. The organ of *seeing* is the *eye*, which is made up of a number of parts, and so wonderfully contrived for admitting and refracting the rays of light, that those which come from the same point of the object, and fall upon different parts of the pupil, are again brought together at the bottom of the eye, and by that means the whole object is painted on a
mem-

membrane called the *retina*, which is spread there

But how is it possible, says Sir *Harry*, for you to know that the object is thus painted on the *retina* ? In some measure from the structure of the eye, replied the Philosopher; but, I think, it is manifest from that disorder of the eye, which surgeons call the *gutta serena*, the very complaint which my Lord's Butler has in one of his eyes. If you examine it you will find that he has no light with that eye, tho' it looks as perfect as the other with which he sees well ; this is, therefore, occasioned by some paralytic, or other disorder in that membrane, or expansion of the optic nerve, which we call the *retina*, and proves that all vision arises from thence.

That which produces in us the sensation which we call Seeing, is *light*, for without *light* nothing is visible. Now light may be considered either as it radiates from luminous bodies directly to our eyes, and thus we see these luminous bodies themselves ; as the *Sun*, a lighted *torch*, &c. or as it is reflected from other bodies, and thus we see a *flower*, a *man*, &c. or a picture reflected from them to our eyes by the rays of light.

It is to be observed that the bodies which respect the light are of three sorts, 1. Those that

that emit the rays of light, as the sun and fixed stars, 2. Those that transmit the rays of light, as the air, and, 3. Those that reflect them, as the moon, the earth, iron, &c. The first we call *luminous*, the second *pellucid*, and the third *opaque* bodies. It is also to be observed, that the rays of light themselves are never seen, but by their means we see the luminous bodies from which they originally came, and the opaque bodies from which they are reflected, thus, for instance, when the moon shines, we cannot see the rays which pass from the sun to the moon; but, by their means, we see the moon from whence they are reflected.

If the eye be placed directly in the medium through which the rays pass to it, the medium is not seen, for we never see the air through which the rays come to our eyes. But if a *pellucid* body, through which the rays are to pass, be placed at a distance from our eye, that body will be seen, as well as those bodies from whence the rays came that pass through it to our eyes, for instance, he who looks through a pair of spectacles not only sees bodies through them, but also sees the glass itself, because the glass, being a solid body, reflects some rays of light from its surface; and being placed at a convenient distance from the eye, may be seen by those reflected rays, at the same time that bodies at a greater distance are seen by the transmitted rays; and this is the reason, perhaps, why objects are seen more distinctly through a reflecting than through a refracting telescope.

There are two kinds of opaque bodies, namely, those that are not *specular*, as the moon, the earth, a man, a horse, &c. and others that are *specular* or *mirrors*, like those in reflecting telescopes, whose surfaces being polished reflect the rays in the same order as they came from other bodies, and show us their images; and rays that are thus reflected from opaque bodies always bring with them to the eye the idea of colour, though this colour in bodies is nothing more than a disposition to reflect to the eye one sort of rays more copiously or in greater plenty than another; for particular rays impress upon the eye particular colours, some are *red*, others *blue, yellow, green*, &c. Now it is to be observed, that every body of light which comes from the Sun seems to be compounded of these various sorts of rays, and as some of them are more *refrangible* than others, that is to say, are more turned out of their course in passing from one medium to

and of his UNDERSTANDING. 107

to another, it necessarily follows that they will be separated after such refraction, and their colours appear distinct. The most refrangible of these are the *violet*, and the least the *red*; the intermediate ones, in order, are *indigo, blue, green, yellow,* and *orange.*

How do you know, Mr. Philosopher, that colours are separated in this manner? says Sir *Harry*, I have no notion of these doctrines without demonstration. That you may have, if you please, replied the Philosopher. Pray, Master *Lovelace,* hand me that Prism.

Now, Sir *Harry,* if you will please to hold this Prism in the beams of the Sun, you will see the colours separated in the manner I have mentioned. Please to look, Lady *Caroline,* the separation is very pleasing, and you will find what I said of the *rainbow* in

K 2 my

my third Lecture confirmed by this experiment.

All these rays differ not only in *refrangibility* but in *reflexibility*; I mean the property of being reflected some more easily than others. And hence arise all the various colours of bodies.

The *whiteness* of the Sun's light is owing, it is supposed, to a mixture of all the original colours in a due proportion, and *whiteness* in other bodies is a disposition to reflect all the colours of light nearly in the same proportion as they are mixed in the original rays of the Sun, as *blackness*, on the contrary, is only a disposition to absorb or stifle, without reflection, most of the rays of every sort that fall on these bodies; and it is for that reason, we may suppose, that *black* clothes are warmer than those of any other colour. The inhabitants of *Naples*, though in so hot a clime, for the most part wear black

Light, as we have already observed, is successively propagated with most amazing swiftness, for it comes from the Sun to the Earth in about seven or eight minutes, though at the distance of seventy millions of miles.

HEARING is the next most extensive of our senses, the organ of which is the *Ear*, whose

whose structure is extremely curious, as may be seen in the books of Anatomy.

That which the ear conveys to the brain is called sound, though till it reaches and affects the perceptive part, it is in reality nothing but motion, and this motion, which produces in us the perception of sound, is a vibration of the air, occasioned by a very short and quick tremulous motion of the body from whence it is propagated. That sound is conveyed in this manner, may be known by what is observed and felt in the strings of musical instruments, and of bells, which tremble or vibrate as long as we perceive any sound come from them, and from this effect which they produce in us, they are called Sounding Bodies.

Sound is propagated at a great rate, but not near so fast as light. I don't know that, says Lady *Caroline*. Then your Ladyship has forgot what passed in our Lecture upon *Air*, replied the Philosopher; and to confirm by experiment what I advanced, I must beg his Lordship to order one of the servants to go a distance into the park, and discharge a *gun*. The Gentlemen were averse to this, it being an observation they had made a hundred times; but to gratify the young people,

people, my Lord ordered his Game-keeper out, and when the piece was discharged, they had the satisfaction of seeing the fire long before they heard the report.

SMELLING is another sense which seems to be excited in us by external bodies, and sometimes by bodies at a great distance; but that which immediately affects the nose, the organ of smelling, and produces in us the sensation of any smell, are effluvia or invisible particles that fly from those bodies to our *olfactory* nerves. How do you prove this, young Gentleman? says Sir *Har*. Sir, replied the Philosopher, had you been here yesterday you would not have asked this question, for, as the wind was North East, the effluvia from my Lord's brick-kilns were ready to suffocate us; but now the wind is turned to the South-West you observe no such thing, because those *effluvia* are driven a contrary way.

The power which some bodies have of emitting these *effluvia* or steams without being visibly diminished, is to me most amazing; yet that it is true we know by abundant experience. A single grain of *musk* will scent a thousand rooms, and send forth these odoriferous particles for a great number of years without being spent. Surely these particles must

must be extremely small; yet their minuteness is nothing when compared with the particles of light, which pervade and find their way through glass, or to the magnetic *effluvia* which pass freely through metallic bodies, whereas those effluvia that produce the sensation of smelling, notwithstanding their wonderful property of scenting all places into which they are brought, and without any sensible diminution, are yet too gross to pass the membranes of a bladder, and many of them will scarce find their way through a common white paper.

There are but few names to express the infinite number of scents that we meet with. I know of none but those of *sweet, stinking, rank, musty,* and *sour,* for so barren is our language in this respect, that the rest are expressed either by degrees of comparison, or from epithets borrowed from bodies that produce scent, which must, in many cases, be very inexpressive, for the smell of a *rose,* of a *violet,* and of *musk,* though all sweet, are as distinct as any scents whatever.

The next sense under our consideration is TASTE, the organ of which is the *tongue,* and the *palate,* but principally the tongue. Ay, and a pretty organ it is, says Lady Carol—. When used to your Ladyship's discretion, Madam, replied the Philosopher. But I must observe to your Ladyship, and the rest of the good company, that though bodies which emit *light*, *sounds*, and *scents*, are seen, heard, and smelt at a distance, yet no bodies can produce taste, without being immediately applied to the organ; for though the meat be placed at your mouth, you know not what taste it will produce till you have touched it with your tongue or palate.

Though there is an amazing variety of tastes, yet here, as in scents, we have but a few general names to express the whole; *sweet*, *sour*, *bitter*, *harsh*, *smooth*, and *rank*, are all that I can recollect; and our other ideas of taste are generally conveyed by borrowed similitudes and expressions by those of *scents*. It is surprising, says the Ambassador, that in this age of gluttony, your language should be so barren as not to afford you words to express those ideas which are excited by exquisite flavours. Sir, says the Marquis, this may be easily accounted for. I must inform your Excellency, that we are indebted for our most expressive terms to the Poets, who were never much acquainted with good eating, and are less so since literature has lost its zest. Very true, my Lord,
says

says Sir *Harry*, their dishes, poor creatures, have lately been of the mental kind; but had you a few rich Poets that could afford to live like people of taste, instead of your sweets and your sours, and such old fashion terms, you would have the *calapash* and *calapee* flavour, the *live-lobster* flavour, the *whipt pig* flavour, and a list of others, as long——as my arm. Fie, Sir *Harry*, says the Marchioness, no more of that, I beg; you know Lady *Caroline* can't bear the name of Barbarity. Nor I neither, says the Ambassador; but pray what barbarity is there in this, Madam? Oh! none at all, replied Sir *Harry*, I only mean to insinuate that some of our great people are not content with having food brought from the *East* and *West Indies*, and every other part of the world, to gratify their palates, but they must roast lobsters alive, and whip young pigs to death to make them tender. Good God! says the Ambassador, are there people in *England* capable of such acts of inhumanity? A man that would do that would murder me, if the law did not stand between us; and the law is but a poor screen where humanity is lost and conscience is lulled to sleep. I'll apply to the King my master for my dismission, and no longer live with a people who have adopted

such

such diabolical customs. The Ambassador was so much in a passion, that it was with difficulty my Lord Marquis pacified him; and poor Lady *Caroline*, whose kind soul sympathizes with every creature in distress, was in tears at the bare rehearsal of these acts of cruelty. Upon which the Baronet was blamed by all the company, except myself, and, I think he never showed so much good sense in his life; for there was one in the room who deserved the reproof.

When the Ambassador had sat down with a sigh, and Lady *Caroline* had wiped the precious pearly drops from her cheeks, our Philosopher arose and thus pursued his Lecture.

I have already taken notice of four of our senses, and am now come to the fifth and last, I mean that of the Touch, which is a sense spread over the whole body, though it is more particularly the business of the hands and fingers; for by them the tangible qualities of bodies are known, since we discover by the *touch* of the fingers, and sometimes, indeed, by the *touch* of other parts of the body, whether things are *hard*, *soft*, *rough*, *smooth*, *wet*, *dry*, &c. But the qualities which most affect this sense are *heat* and *cold*, and which, indeed, are the great

engines

Chariot fired by Motion

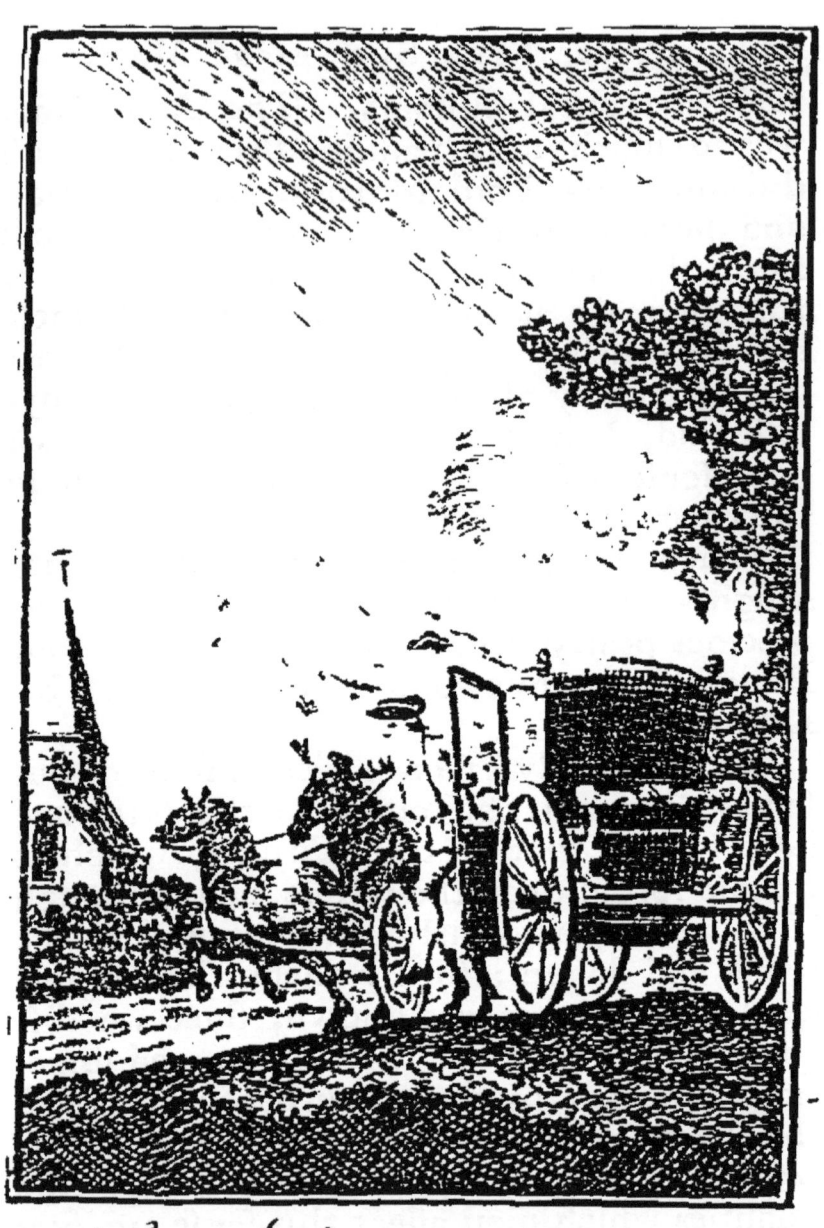

engines of Nature, for by a due temperament of those two opposite qualities most of her productions are formed.

What we call *heat* is occasioned by the agitation of the insensible parts of the body that produces in us that sensation; and when the parts of a body are violently agitated, we say, and indeed we feel, that body is *hot*, so that that which to our sensation is *heat*, in the object is nothing but *motion*. Hey-day, says Lady *Caroline*, what sort of Philosophy is this? Why, Madam, says Sir *Harry*, this is a position which has been laid down by these airy Gentlemen for a long time, but which never has been proved by experiment. Take care, Baronet, says the Marquis, or you'll forfeit all pretensions to Philosophy. The forfeiture, my Lord, is made already, says the Philosopher; Sir *Harry* has been bold enough to deny that which experience every day confirms for truth. If what we call Heat is not motion, or occasioned by the motion of bodies, how came my Lord's mill to take fire the other day, when it was running round without a proper supply of corn? And how came your post chariot to fire while running down *Breakneck hill*, Sir *Harry*? Consider, there was nobody with a torch under the axle-tree;

tree; but this is a part of philosophy known even to the poor ignorant *Indians*, who, when hunting at a great distance from home, and wanting fire to dress their meat, take a bow and a string and rub two pieces of wood together till they produce flame. But you may see, Sir *Harry*, that heat is occasioned by the motion of bodies, by only rubbing this piece of smooth brass on the table—stay, I'll rub it—It must be done briskly. There, now you'll feel it hot; but cease this motion for a time, and the brass will become cold again, whence we may infer, that as heat is nothing but the insensible particles of bodies put into motion, so cold, on the contrary, is occasioned by the cessation of the motion of those particles, or their being placed in a state of rest.

But bodies appear *hot* or *cold* in proportion to the temperament of that part of the human body to which they are applied, so that what seems hot to one, may not seem so to another. This is so true, that the same body felt by the two hands of the same man, may at the same instant of time appear warm to the one hand and cold to the other, if with the one hand he has been rubbing any thing, while the other was kept in a state of rest; and for no other reason but because

the

the motion of the infensible particles of that hand with which he has been rubbing, will be more brisk than the particles of the other which was at rest.

I have mentioned those objects which are peculiar to each of our senses, as *light* and *colour* to the *sight*; *sound* to the *hearing*; *odours* to the *smell*, &c. but there are two others common to all the senses, which deserve our notice, and these are *pleasure* and *pain*, which the senses may receive by their own peculiar objects, for we know that a proper portion of light is pleasing, but that too much offends the eye; some sounds delight, while others are disagreeable, and grate the ear; so heat, in a moderate degree, is very pleasant; yet that heat may be so increased as to give the most intolerable pain. But these things are too well known to be longer insisted on.

Now from the *ideas* or *conceptions* formed in the mind, by means of our senses, and the operations of the mind itself, are laid the foundation of the human understanding, the lowest degree of which is *perception*; and to conceive a right notion of this, we must distinguish the first objects of it, which are *simple ideas*, such as are represented by the words, *red, blue, bitter, sweet,* &c. from
the

the other objects of our senses; to which we may add the internal operations of our own minds, or the objects of reflection, such as are *thinking, willing,* &c. for all our ideas are first obtained by *sensation* and *reflection.* The mind having gained variety of *simple ideas,* by putting them together, forms what are called *compounded* or *complex ideas,* as those signified by the words, *man, horse, marygold, windmill,* &c.

The next operation of the mind (or of the understanding) in its progress to knowledge, is that of abstracting its ideas; for by abstraction they are made general; and a *general idea* is to be considered as separated from time and place, and lodged in the mind to represent any particular thing that is conformable to it.

Knowledge, which is the highest degree of the speculative faculties, consists in the perception of the truth of affirmative or negative propositions; and this perception is either immediate or mediate. When, by comparing two ideas together in the mind, we perceive their agreement or disagreement, as that black is not white; that the whole is bigger than a part; and that two and two are equal to four, &c. it is called immediate perception, or *intuitive* knowledge; and as
the

the truth of these and the like propositions is so evident as to be known by a simple intuition of the ideas themselves, they are also called *self-evident propositions*.

Mediate perception is when the agreement or disagreement of two ideas is made known by the intervention of some other ideas: Thus if it be affirmed that my Lord's bay horse is as high as my father's, the agreement or disagreement may be seen by applying the same measure to both: And this is called *demonstration*, or *rational knowledge*. The dimensions of any two bodies which cannot be brought together, may be thus known, by the same measure being applied to them both.

But the understanding is not confined to certain truth; it also judges of *probability*, which consists in the *likely* agreement or disagreement of ideas, and the assenting to any proposition as probable, is called *opinion*, or *belief*.—We have now finished this Course of Lectures. I hope not, says Lady *Caroline*, with some emotion!—Why, Madam, returned the Philosopher, we have taken a cursory view of natural bodies, and their causes and effects; which I have endeavoured to explain in such a manner as to be intelligible, at least, if not entertaining; and pray what more did your Ladyship expect? Sir, replied the Lady, I am greatly pleased with the account you have given us, and I thank you, Sir, for the pains you have taken to answer the many questions I have troubled you with. What I had further to hope, was, that you would have given us, when you was on the subject of Animals, some strictures on the cruelty with which they are too often treated; and have thrown in reflections and observations tending to inforce in mankind a different conduct. This I wished for, and should have been glad to have had Sir *Thomas* and his Lady here at the same time; who are both extremely fond of their little domestic creatures, and I admire them for their tenderness and compassion. These feelings and sentiments of the human heart, Madam, says the Philosopher, add much to the dignity of our nature, and I am greatly delighted with such behaviour, but I am afraid Lady *Caroline*, that we often mistake characters of this kind, and take that for humanity and tenderness, which is only the effect of fancy or self-love. That Sir *Thomas* has compassion, I grant you, but I am afraid it is only for himself. He loves his dogs and horses, because his dogs and horses give him pleasure, but to other creatures that afford him none, he is absolutely infensible. I have seen him even at *Christmas*, feed his pretty *pupps*, as he calls them, with delicacies; but rave at the same time, in a merciless manner, at poor children who were shivering at his gate, and send them away empty handed. Our neighbour, Sir *William*, is also of the same disposition; he will not sell a horse that is declining, for fear he should fall into the hands of a master who might treat him with cruelty; but he is largely concerned in the slave trade, (which, I think is carried on by none but *we good Christians*, to the dishonour of our *cœlestial Master)* and makes no difficulty of separating the husband from the wife, the parents from the children, and all of them (as well as our own people, who are procured by his *crimps,)* from their native country, to be sold in a foreign market, like so many horses, and often to the most merciless of the human race. I remember him in great distress for his pointer *Phillis*, who had lost her *puppies*; but the same afternoon I saw him, without the least compunction of mind, press a poor man into the sea service, and tear him from his wife and children, for no other *crime*, but because he had fought bravely for his King and country in the last war, and being now settled in business, in business, and having a family, did not chuse to enter the service again. Is this humanity, Madam? Is this morality? But above all, is this Christianity? And are these the blessed effects of the liberty we boast of?—I don't expect a reply, Lady *Caroline*, for I shall have occasion to say much more on these subjects in my next Course of Lectures, and then, perhaps, you will honour me with your observations. But in the mean time don't let us be misled by specious pretences. We cannot judge of any man, Madam, by one single action, but by the tenour and result of all his actions, and this requires deep penetration and an intimate knowledge of human life.

Benevolence, Lady *Caroline*, should be universal, for it is an emanation of the Supreme Being, whose mercy and goodness are extended to all his creatures; as ours also should be, for they are fellow tenants with us of the globe we inhabit.

I have often thought, Madam, that most of the mischiefs which embarrass society, and render one man contemptible to another, are owing to inordinate *ambition* or extreme love of *power*, and of *wealth*, the means by which it is procured, for all the gold a man possesses, beyond that portion which is requisite

quisite for himself and family, only serves to inflame his ambition; as all the wine we drink, more than is necessary to recruit the drooping spirits, answers no other purpose but to intoxicate the mind.

I have seen a book, Lady *Caroline*, in my Papa's library, which gives some account of one *Lycurgus*, an old *Grecian* Lawgiver, with whose character you ought to be acquainted —— This man, Madam, was of opinion, that religion, virtue, and good manners, were the only natural cements and preservation of liberty, peace, and friendship, which he found had been destroyed and extirpated by means of wealth and self-interest; he therefore prohibited the use of gold and silver, and of all kinds of luxury in the state, and established such a plan for the education of youth of every denomination, as was most likely to confirm and habituate them in the practise of religion and virtue, and secure to the *Spartans* and their posterity the blessings of liberty and peace.

The event proved that his institutions were founded on sound policy, and a perfect knowledge of human nature: for in the space of five hundred years, that is to say, from the time of *Lycurgus* to the introduction of wealth into the state by *Lysander*, in the reign of the first *Agis*, there was no mutiny among the people; every man submitted chearfully to the laws of *Lycurgus*, and all were so united and powerful in consequence of their virtue, sobriety, and the martial discipline he had established, (which was that of a national militia,) that *Sparta*, a very small inconsiderable state, not only gave laws to the rest of *Greece*, but made even the *Persian* Monarchs tremble, though masters of the richest and most extensive empire in the world. But when this great and virtuous people of *Sparta* had conquered *Athens*, and from thence introduced wealth and luxury into their own country, they lost their virtue, dwindled to nothing, and were themselves enslaved. Nor is this a matter of wonder; for where Religion and Virtue are set at a distance, and Wealth leads the way to posts of honour and trust, some people will stick at nothing to obtain gold; but were dignities of this kind conferred on the most deserving, and none but men of virtue and superior abilities promoted to places of trust and power, there would be no frauds in the State, or violence among the People, and we might then hope to enjoy the felicities of the *Golden Age*.

Man in that age no rule but Reason knew,
And with a native bent did good pursue;
Unaw'd by punishment, and void of fear,
His words were simple and his soul sincere.
By no *forc'd laws* his passions were confin'd,
For *Conscience* kept his heart, and calm'd his mind,
Peace o'er the world her blessed sway maintain'd,
And e'en in Deserts smiling *Plenty* reign'd.

F I N I S.

ADVERTISEMENT.

⁎ The Author of the preceding Sheets has in most Places explained the technical Terms, but in all he could not, without increasing the volume beyond the Size intended, or destroying the Thread of the Narration, he would, therefore, recommend the occasional use of some good Dictionary, by turning to which the Terms will be so fixed in the young Student's Mind, that he will seldom be at a Loss in reading any other Treatise on philosophical Subjects.—Mention is made of the *Pocket Dictionary*, (Page 95) not because the Terms are better defined in that Book than any other, but because it is sold only for *Three Shillings* bound, and by being contracted into less Compass than any other Dictionaries, is rendered more portable and convenient for the Pocket

To the PARENTS, GUARDIANS, and GOVERNESSES, in *Great-Britain, Ireland,* and the *British Colonies.*

AT a Time when all complain of the Depravity of Human Nature, and the Degeneracy of the present Age, any Design that is calculated to mend the Heart, and inforce a contrary Conduct, must surely claim the Attention and Encouragement of the Public.

It has been said, and very wisely, that the only way to remedy these Evils, is to begin with the rising Generation, and to take the Mind in its Infant State, when it is uncorrupted and susceptible of any Impression, to represent to Children their Duties and future Interests in a Manner that shall seem rather intended to amuse than instruct, to excite their Attention with Images and Pictures that are familiar and pleasing; and to warm their Affections with such little Histories as are capable of giving them Delight and of impressing on their tender Minds proper Sentiments of Religion, Justice, Honour, and Virtue.

When Infant Reason grows apace it cal's
For the kind Hand of an assiduous Care;
Delightful Task! To rear the tender Thought,
To teach the young Idea how to shoot,
To pour the fresh Instruction o'er the Mind,
To breathe th' inspiring Spirit, and to fix
The generous Purpose in the glowing Breast.
                              THOMSON.

How far Mr. NEWBERY's little Books may tend to forward this good Work, may be, in some Measure, seen by what are already published, and, it is presumed, will more evidently appear by others which are coming from the Press.

Books for the Instruction and Amusement of Children, printed for T. CARNAN, *Successor to* Mr. J. NEWBERY, *in* St. Paul's Church-yard, London.

1. THE Renowned History of *Giles Gingerbread*, a little Boy who lived upon Learning. Price *One Penny*, adorned with Cuts.

2. *Nurse Truelove's Christmas Box*; or the *Golden Play Thing* for little Children: by which they may learn the Letters as soon as they can speak, and know how to behave, so as to make every Body love them. Adorned with 30 Cuts. Price *One Penny*.

3. *Tom Thumb*'s Folio; or, a New Penny Plaything for little Giants. To which is prefixed, an Abstract of the Life of Mr. Thumb; and an historical Account of the wonderful Deeds he performed, together with some Anecdotes respecting Grumbo

the Great Giant. Adorned with Cuts. Price *One Penny.*

4. *Entertaining Fables* for the Instruction of Children; embellished with Cuts. Price *One Penny.*

5. The *London Cries*, for the Amusement of all the good Children throughout the World. Taken from the Life. Price 1 *d.*

6. The *Lilliputian Auction.* To which all little Masters and Misses are invited, by Charley Chatter. Price *One Penny.*

7. The *Lilliputian Masquerade*; recommended to the Perusal of those Sons and Daughters of Folly the Frequenters of the Pantheon, Almack's, and Cornelly's. Embellished with Cuts, for the Instruction and Amusement of the rising Generation. Price of a Subscription Ticket, not *Two Guineas*, but *Two Pence.*

8. *Nurse Truelove's New Year's Gift:* or, The Book of Books for Children. Adorned with Cuts, and designed for a Present to every little Boy who would become a great Man, and ride upon a fine Horse, and to every little Girl who would become a great Woman, and ride in a Lord Mayor's gilt Coach. Price *Two Pence.*

9. The *Easter Gift*; or, The way to be very Good. *A Book very much wanted.* Adorned with Cuts. Price *Two Pence.*

in *St. Paul's Church Yard.* 129

10 The *Whitsuntide Gift*; or, The Way to be very Happy. *A Book necessary for all Families.* Embellished with Cuts. Price *Two Pence.*

11. The Little *Lottery Book* for Children, containing a new Method of playing them into a Knowledge of the Letters, Figures, &c. Embellished with above Fifty Cuts, and published with the Approbation of the Court of Common Sense. Price *Two Pence.*

12. A *Pretty Plaything* for Children of all Denominations: Containing, I. The Alphabet in Verse, for the Use of little Children. II. An Alphabet in Prose, interspersed with proper Lessons in Life, for the Use of great Children. III. Tom Noddy and his Sister Sue, a Lilliputian Story. IV. The sound of the Letters explained by visible Objects, delineated on Copper Plates. V. The Cuz's Chorus, set to Music; to be sung by Children, in order to teach them to join their Letters in Syllables, and pronounce them properly. The whole embellished with variety of Cuts after the Manner of Ptolemy. Price *Two Pence* bound.

13. The *Royal Battledore*; or, First Book for Children. Price *Two Pence.*

14. The *Royal Primer*; or, An easy and pleasant Guide to the Art of Reading. Interspersed

M

terspersed with a great variety of short and diverting Stories, with suitable Morals and Reflections. Adorned with Twenty-seven Cuts. Price *Three Pence* bound.

15. A little pretty *Pocket Book*, intended for the Instruction and Amusement of little Master *Tommy*, and pretty Miss *Polly*; with Two Letters from *Jack the Giant Killer*, concerning a Ball and Pincushion, the use of which will infallibly make *Tommy* a good Boy, and *Polly* a good Girl. To which is added a little *Song Book*. being a new Attempt to teach Children the Use of the English Alphabet, by way of Diversion. Price bound *Three Pence*.

16. The *Mother's Gift*, or a Present for all little Children who are good. Embellished with Cuts. Price *Three Pence*.

17. The *Fairing*; or, Golden Toy for Children.

    In which they may see all the Fun in the Fair,
    And at Home be as happy as if they were there.

A Book of great Consequence to all whom it may concern. Price *Sixpence* bound, and Adorned with Cuts.

18. The renowned History of little *Goody Two Shoes*, afterwards called Mrs. *Margery Two Shoes*; with the Means by which she acquired

acquired her Learning and Wisdom, and in Consequence thereof, her Estate. Price *Sixpence*, bound and adorned with Cuts.

19. The *Infant Tutor*; or an easy Spelling Book for little Masters and Misses. Made pleasing, with variety of Stories and Fables. Embellished with Cuts. Price *Sixpence* bound.

20. Be *Merry and Wise*; or the Cream of the *Jest* and *Marrow* of *Maxims*, for the Conduct of Life. Published for the Use of all little good Boys and Girls, by *T. Trapwit*, Esq. adorned with Cuts. Price *Sixpence* bound.

———*Would you be agreeable in Company, and useful to Society, carry some merry Jests in your Mind, and honest Maxims in your Heart.* GROTIUS.

21. *Fables in Verse*, for the Improvement of the Young and the Old, by *Abraham Æsop*, Esq. to which are added, FABLES in *Verse* and *Prose*, with the Conversation of Birds and Beasts, at their several Meetings, Routs, and Assemblies. By *Woglog*, the great Giant. Illustrated with a variety of curious Cuts, and an Account of the Lives of the Authors. Price *Sixpence* bound.

22. The

132　Books printed for *T. Carnan*,

22. The *Holy Bible* abridged. or, The History of the Old and New Testament; illustrated with Notes, and adorned with Cuts, for the Use of Children. Price 6 *d.* bound.—*Suffer little Children to come unto me, and forbid them not.* St. Luke

23. A Collection of *Pretty Poems*, for the Amusement of Children Three Feet high. By *Thomas Tagg*, Esq. Adorned with above Sixty Cuts. Price *Sixpence* bound.

24. A New *History* of *England*, from the Invasion of *Julius Cæsar* to the Reign of King George II. Adorned with the Cuts of all the Kings and Queens who have reigned since the Norman Conquest. Price *Sixpence* bound ——*The Memory of Things past ought not to be extinguished by Length of Time, nor great and memorable Actions remain destitute of Glory.* Herodotus.

25. The *Valentine's Gift:* or, The whole History of *Valentine's Day*; containing the Way to preserve *Truth, Honour,* and *Integrity* unshaken. *Very necessary in a trading Nation.* Price *Sixpence* bound.

26. The *Little Female Orators:* or, Nine Evenings Entertainment; with Observations. Embellished with Cuts. Price *Sixpence.*

27. Letters

27. Letters between *Master Tommy* and *Miss Nancy Goodwill*. Containing the History of their Holyday Amusements. With Cuts. Price *Sixpence*.

28. The *Pretty Book* for Children. or, An Easy Guide to the English Tongue; designed for the Instruction of those who cannot read, as well as for the Entertainment of those that can. Price 6d. bound.

29. A *Pretty Book of Pictures* for little Masters and Misses or, *Tommy Trip*'s History of Birds and Beasts; with a familiar Description of each in Verse and Prose. To which is added, the History of little *Tom Trip* himself, of his Dog *Jowler*, and of *Woglog*, the great Giant. Price *Sixpence* bound.

30. *Food for the Mind*. or, a New *Riddle Book*; compiled for the Use of the great and little good Boys and Girls of *England*, *Scotland*, and *Ireland*. By *John the Giant Killer*, Esq. Adorned with Cuts. Price *Sixpence*.

31. The wonderful Life and surprizing Adventures of that renowned Hero *Robinson Crusoe*, who lived twenty eight Years in an uninhabited Island, which he afterwards colonized. Embellished with Cuts. Price *Sixpence*.

134 Books printed for *T. Carnan*,

32. *Sixpennyworth of Wit* or, Little Stories for little Folks of all Denominations. Adorned with Cuts.

33. Alphabet Royal ou Guide commode et agreeable dans l'Art de Lire. Le Prix seulement 6d.

34. The *Royal Psalter*, or King David's Meditations: to which is added at the Bottom of each Page, Rational Meditation; on moral and divine Subjects, instructive and entertaining to both young and old; and at the Beginning of each Psalm a short Explanation thereof. Adapted to the Use of Schools as well as private Families. Price A sixpence bound.

35. *A Easy Guide* to the *English Language*, in two Parts. Part I. Contains, 1. Tables of Words from one to nine Syllables, with Lessons properly adapted to each Table; also select Maxims, calculated to imprint upon the tender Minds of Youth the Principles of Wisdom, while they are yet but learning the Rudiments of Speech. 2. Of Words of the same Sound, but differing in Sense 3. Of Contractions for the readier Dispatch of Business. 4. Forms of Address to Persons of distinguished Rank, as well as to those in common Life. Part II. contains,

contains, 1. A plain and familiar Grammar, by way of Question and Answer, for the Use, not only of the English Scholar, but of those who intend to learn the Latin Tongue; as it will give them distinct Notions of the different Parts of Speech, and the Agreement of Words; and thereby greatly facilitate their Progress. 2. Sentences and Maxims, selected from the Writings and Observations of Philosophers, and other wise Men; proper to exercise and improve the Memory. 3. Select Fables, with proper Pictures, designed as an Amusement to young Beginners, and to caution them against cunning and deceitful Persons. 4. Forms of Prayer, proper for Children, on every Occasion. Price *One Shilling* bound.

36. A set of *Fifty six Squares*, and Directions for playing with them, so contrived as to learn Children to read in a little Time, and to yield them as much Entertainment as any of their Play Games usually do By which Means, a great deal of Time commonly idled away by Children, will be profitably as well as plentifully applied; upon the Plan of the great Mr. *Locke*. Price *One Shilling.*

37. The

37. The *Lilliputian Magazine:* or, The Young Gentleman and Lady's Golden Library. Being an Attempt to mend the World, to render the Society of Man more amiable, and to establish the Plainness, Simplicity, Wisdom, and Virtue of the Golden Age, so much celebrated by the Poets and Historians. Adorned with Cuts. Price *One Shilling* bound.

38. A Collection of Pretty Poems, for the Amusement of Children Six Feet high, interspersed with a series of Letters from Cousin *Sam* to Cousin *Sue*, on the Subjects of Criticism, Poetry, and Politics, with Notes Variorum. Calculated with a Design to do good; and adorned with a Variety of Copper-plate Cuts by the best Masters. Price bound *One Shilling*.

39. *Short Histories* for the Improvement of the Mind. Extracted chiefly from the Works of the celebrated *Joseph Addison*, Esq. Sir *Richard Steele*, Mr *Rollin*, and other eminent Writers; with suitable *Reflections* by the Editor. Price *One Shilling*.

40. The *Museum* for young Gentlemen and Ladies; or, a Compleat Tutor for little Masters and Misses. Price *One Shilling* bound.

41. The

41. The *New Testament*, adapted to the Capacities of Children, or, the *Four Gospels* harmonized and adorned with Copper-Plate Cuts. To which is prefixed a Preface, setting forth the Nature and Necessity of the Work. Price *One Shilling*.

42. The *History* of the Life, Actions, Sufferings, and Death of our Blessed Saviour *Jesus Christ*. To which is added the Life of the blessed Virgin *Mary*. Adorned with Copper-plate Cuts. Price *One Shilling* bound.

43. An *History* of the Lives, Actions, Travels, Sufferings, and Death of the *Apostles* and *Evangelists*. Adorned with Copper-plate Cuts. Price *One Shilling* bound.

44. An *History* of the Lives, Travels, Sufferings and Deaths of the Fathers of the *Cristian Church* for the first *Four Centuries*. Adorned with Copper plate Cuts. Price *One Shilling* bound.

45 A *plain* and *concise Exposition* of the Book of *Common Prayer*, with an Account of the *Feasts* and *Festivals*. To which are prefixed, the Lives of the *Compilers* of the *Common Prayer*. Adorned with Copper-plate Cuts. Price *One Shilling*.

46. The *Twelfth-Day Gift*. or, the Grand Exhibition. Containing a curious Collection

Collection of Pieces in Prose and Verse (many of them Originals) which were delivered to a numerous and polite Audience, on the important Subjects of Religion, Morality, History, Philosophy, Policy, Prudence, and Œconomy, at the most noble the Marquis of *Setstar's*, by a Society of young Gentlemen and Ladies, and registered at their Request, by their old Friend Mr. *Newbery*. With which are intermixed some occasional Reflections, and a Narrative, containing the Characters and Behaviour of the several Persons concerned. Price *One Shilling* bound.

47. The *Important Pocket Book*, or the *Valentine's Ledger*, for the Use of those who would live happily in this World and in the next. Price *One Shilling*.

48. The *Words of the Wise*. Designed for the Entertainment and Instruction of younger Minds.

The Wise shall inherit Glory but Shame shall be the Promotion of Fools. Prov. Sol. Price *One Shilling* sewed

49 An *Easy Spelling Dictionary*, (on a new Plan) for the Use of young Gentlemen, Ladies, and Foreigners — In which each Word is accented to prevent a vicious Pronunciation; the several Syllables are pointed by a small Figure in the Margin, and whatever

ever Part of Speech it is, specified by a Letter immediately following each Word. So contrived as to take up no more room in the Pocket than a common Snuff-box, tho' a Companion infinitely more useful. Price bound *One Shilling*.

50 *Letters* on the most common as well as important Occasions in Life: By *Cicero, Pliny, Voiture, Balzac, St. Evremond, Locke,* Lords *Lansdowne, Oxford, Peterborough,* and *Bolingbroke,* Sir *William Temple,* Sir *William Trumbull, Dryden, Atterbury, Garth, Addison, Steele, Pope, Gay, Swift, Berkeley, Rowe,* and other Writers of distinguished Merit; with many Original Letters and Cards by the Editor. Who has also prefixed, a Dissertation on the Epistolary Stile; with proper Directions for addressing Persons of Rank and Eminence. Price 1s. 6d.

51. A Voyage round the *World*, in His Majesty's Ship the *Dolphin*, commanded by the Honourable Commodore *Byron*; in which is contained, a faithful Account of the several Places, People, Plants, Animals, &c. seen on the Voyage. And, among other Particulars, a minute and exact Description of the Streights of Magellan, and of the gigantic People called Patagonians. Together with an accurate Account of seven

Islands

140   Books printed for *T. Carnan*.

Islands lately discovered in the South Seas. By an Officer on Board the said Ship. Price *One Shilling* sewed.

52. A Compendious *History* of the *World*, from the Creation to the Dissolution of the Roman Republic, 2 vols. Price *One Shilling* and *Sixpence* bound.

53. The *Circle* of the *Sciences*, in 7 vols. Price *Seven Shillings*. Containing, Vol. 1. Grammar.—Vol. 2. Arithmetic.—Vol. 3. Rhetoric.—Vol. 4. Poetry.—Vol. 5. Logic. —Vol. 6. Geography.—Vol. 7. Chronology.

54. A Compendious *History* of *England*, from the Invasion by the Romans to the present Time. Adorned with a Map of Great Britain and Ireland, and embellished with 31 Cuts of all the Kings and Queens who have reigned since the Conquest. Price *Two Shillings* bound.

55. An Account of the *Constitution* and present *State* of *Great Britain*; together with a View of its Trade, Policy and Interest respecting other Nations: and of the Curiosities of Great Britain and Ireland. Adorned with Copper-plate Cuts, neatly engraved. Price *Two Shillings* and *Sixpence* bound.